COACHES' GUIDE TO PERFORMANCE-ENHANCING SUPPLEMENTS

D1518875

Nicholas A. Ratamess, Ph.D., CSCS*D

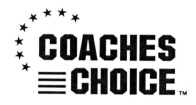

COACHES CHOICE™

ISBN: 1-58518-986-3
Library of Congress Control Number: 2006929423
Book layout: Deborah Oldenburg
Cover design: Studio J Art & Design

Coaches Choice
P.O. Box 1828
Monterey, CA 93942
www.coacheschoice.com

Dedication

This book is dedicated to my wife, Alison, my children, Jessica and Vinnie, and my parents, Nick and Veronica, for their love and support.

Acknowledgments

I want to thank Dr. Jim Peterson and all of the staff at Coaches Choice for their assistance with this book. I want to thank all of my colleagues who I have had the privilege of working with over the years for their inspiration and the knowledge I've gained through their vast expertise in sport ergogenics. I want to thank Dr. William Kraemer for his guidance and my colleagues Drs. Jay Hoffman, Avery Faigenbaum, and Jie Kang for their feedback on the book. In addition, I want to thank my students Michael Loginow and April James for their assistance with some of the photos used in this book.

Contents

1

Sport Supplement Basics

t is virtually impossible to go into a health-food store and not see a wide variety of nutritional supplements available for purchase. Supplements are available in all sizes, brands, and mixtures, leaving coaches in a potential maze of confusion. In fact, it has been estimated that more than 600 dietary supplement manufacturers are located in the United States alone, producing more than 4,000 products totaling annual sales in excess of $4 billion. Which of these supplements should you encourage your athletes to consume? This question is of major concern throughout athletics and may put you in a serious quandary. On one hand, you want each athlete to perform to his maximum potential, which requires optimizing the three major components of success: proper training, recovery, and nutrition. Certainly, the difference between a win and loss, or between first place and fifth place, will depend upon your athletes' strength, muscular and cardiovascular endurance, body composition (i.e., the amount of body fat and muscle mass), power, skill and technique, speed, and agility—all of which are affected by dietary nutrient intake. On the other hand, you also need to be concerned about critical elements such as the cost of supplements, potential side effects or negative health ramifications, ethics, and the potential for a failed drug test due to the intake of certain supplements.

In 1994, Congress passed the Dietary Supplement Health and Education Act (DSHEA). This document defines a supplement as "a product (other than tobacco) intended to supplement the diet that bears or contains one or more of the following dietary ingredients: a vitamin, a mineral, an herb or other botanical, an amino acid, a dietary substance for use by man to supplement the diet by increasing the total daily intake, or a concentrate, metabolite, constituent, extract, or combination of these ingredients." Although this document highlights the importance of supplements for improving health and reducing the risk factors for disease—as well as the importance of the supplement industry as an integral part of the economy—it also made it easier for supplement manufacturers to market their products. Prior to this document, federal legislation passed in 1993 limited the jurisdiction of the Food and Drug Administration (FDA) for regulating the quality, safety, and testing of nutrition supplements. The resulting situation—a combination of marketing ease and a lack of regulation—has contributed to the dramatic increase in sport-supplement marketing and sales.

With the wealth of supplement information available, what do you need to know to properly instruct your athletes? Several key questions are addressed in this chapter that give you an overview of the supplementation process:

- How are supplements classified?
- Do athletes get their optimal nutrient requirements from diet alone?
- Can supplements provide additional benefits beyond what is provided by the diet?
- What is the physiological relevance of a supplement?
- Are supplement labels accurately represented?
- Does the cost of supplements outweigh the benefits?
- Should the age and the training experience of the athlete influence the decision to use nutrition supplements?
- Is supplementation popular among athletes?
- Does the supplement get to where it needs to be in the body?
- Does a dose-response pattern of improvement exist with supplementation?
- Should supplements be taken individually or do they work better when taken in conjunction with other supplements?
- Can supplements be toxic when taken in doses far exceeding the recommended range?
- Does a "placebo" effect exist?
- What are responders and nonresponders?
- Is supplementation ethical?

General Classes of Supplements

Supplements are classified based on their functions in the human body. *Macronutrients* are those nutrients required in large amounts from a person's diet and include proteins, carbohydrates, fats, and water, which makes up approximately 60 to 70 percent of a person's body weight. Proteins are made up of building blocks called amino acids, which have functions both individually and collectively. Some amino acid–related compounds also play key roles in cellular processes, and some show potential ergogenic benefits.

Micronutrients are needed in much smaller amounts in the human diet, but, nevertheless, perform life-sustaining functions in the body. Micronutrients include vitamins and minerals.

Prohormones—which are, in fact, hormones—are precursor molecules involved ultimately in the biosynthesis of testosterone. The legality of obtaining prohormones without a prescription was challenged in 2004.

Cellular metabolism supplements perform multiple functions in skeletal muscle, such as acid-base buffering, energy production, material transport, and volumizing (i.e., increasing the solute concentration such as creatine phosphate within the cells). These supplements may also be included within other multipurpose supplements.

Thermogenic supplements increase metabolism. By increasing the metabolism, an individual can achieve body-fat reductions and possibly affect acute performance, depending on the compound in question (e.g., some thermogenic molecules may impact strength, endurance, and mental focus during exercise).

Antioxidants help control the damaging effects of free radicals on cells in the body. There are a number of nutrients that function as antioxidants, and these act collectively to reduce tissue damage and promote health.

Other supplements have been classified in more general terms. For example, weight-gain, weight-loss, and recovery supplements typically contain multiple nutrients that perform similar functions. *Weight-gain powders and drinks* typically contain high-calorie mixtures of macronutrients, as well as fortification with vitamins and minerals. *Weight-loss supplements* may contain thermogenic compounds, which are micronutrients involved in fat-burning or energy-producing reactions, and appetite suppressants, as well as other cofactors and micronutrients. Multipurpose supplements contain combinations of compounds that may enhance more than one aspect of performance. For example, *recovery supplements* may include large concentrations of carbohydrates, proteins, and some micronutrients, but may also include creatine, ß-hydroxy-ß-methylbutyrate (HMB), antioxidants, glutamine, and other compounds that improve physical function by different means. In addition, pharmacological agents (which require a prescription or may be banned by sport-governing bodies) are also common.

Nutrient Deficiency

A deficiency indicates a lack of, or a suboptimal intake of, one or more nutrients that are essential to optimal bodily function. Supplementation can play an important role in correcting nutrient deficiencies in athletes who have poor diets and/or who fail to take into account the greater nutrient requirements of heavy training. Some athletes may be

- Protein, amino acid, and amino-acid derivatives

- Carbohydrate

- Fat

- Weight gain

- Vitamin

- Mineral

- Herbal

- Thermogenic and weight loss

- Cell metabolism

- Pharmacological

- Miscellaneous

Figure 1-1. General classes of supplements

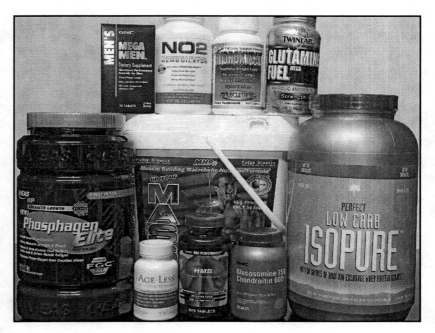

Figure 1-2. Various types of supplements

deficient in certain macro- or micronutrients, and supplementation can help correct these deficiencies. With the rigors of off- and in-season training, practice, and competition, the nutrient needs of an athlete are far greater than those of a nonathlete. If these needs are not met, the athlete may be at a disadvantage.

It is important to note that nutrients work in synergy. In other words, for one nutrient to function properly, balance must be attained among other nutrients that perform similar functions or are involved in the same reaction. For example, vitamins and minerals serve as cofactors in bodily reactions. Because multiple vitamins or minerals are involved in certain reactions, a deficiency in only one can limit the process or slow down the reactions. A common example is vitamin E and selenium, as these micronutrients work in synergy as antioxidants. Therefore, supplements that correct deficiencies can enhance performance, but they are not truly ergogenic because they would provide no further benefit if dietary intake was adequate.

To achieve adequate dietary intake of all essential nutrients, athletes must increase the amount of food and beverages they consume. This task may be difficult, especially during the midst of a heavy training, practice, and competition schedule. Additional time constraints from school and/or work may also exist, thereby causing the athlete some degree of difficulty in maintaining a consistent meal plan. Training, practice, and competition, especially in hot, humid weather, have the additional antagonizing effect of reducing the athlete's appetite. When taking all of these variables into consideration, the difficulty facing an athlete when trying to consume sufficient macro- and micronutrients solely from the diet becomes more evident. This scenario provides an example of when supplementation gives an athlete a competitive edge.

The ability to consume nutrients from nonfood sources becomes important for preventing a deficiency. Sports supplements provide another practical advantage for athletes. Because many sports supplements are available in liquid or powder form (where the powder is mixed into a liquid drink) or as health bars, they provide essential nutrients rapidly and with great flexibility of consumption (i.e., they can easily be transported or consumed any time of day, including those times when the athlete is in class, at work, etc., and may have limited access to food). In addition, sport-supplement drinks can quench thirst and rehydrate athletes during training, practice, and competition. They are more easily digestible than a meal, which gives the athlete quicker access to nutrients. Therefore, sports supplements provide several advantages to athletes in the quest to minimize the risk of nutritional deficiency.

Ergogenic Supplements

The term "ergogenic" refers to performance or work enhancement. It originates from the Greek *ergon* (meaning work) and *gennan* (meaning to produce). In supplement terms, a chemical compound that enhances performance beyond that of normal dietary intake of that compound is considered ergogenic. By this definition, an ergogenic supplement should enhance some facet of performance when no nutrient deficiency is observed. Ergogenic supplements may:

- Increase muscle strength and power
- Increase muscle size
- Increase muscular endurance and reduce fatigue
- Enhance immune-system function and recovery between workouts
- Increase energy availability and reduce body fat
- Improve specific parameters of sports performance

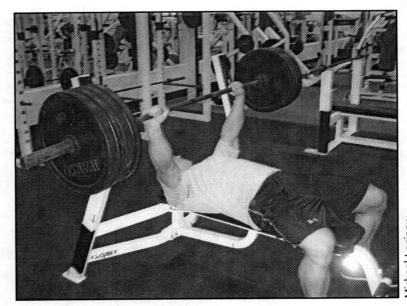

Figure 1-3. A strength-trained athlete

Michael Loginow

Many supplement labels claim that product to be ergogenic. Manufacturers of nutrition supplements have as their sole purpose the marketing and selling of their products. Therefore, exaggerated claims are not uncommon. You must be aware of unsubstantiated claims that may tempt an athlete to purchase a supplement. Additional scientific studies are needed to properly investigate the ergogenic potential of supplement use. Sport scientists carefully design studies by doing the following:

- Standardizing the athletes' diets during the study to isolate the effects of the supplement

- Using a placebo (i.e., a "fake" supplement) as a control in such as way that neither the investigator nor the athlete knows what is being taken (to avoid bias)
- Administering precise doses of the supplement to the athletes
- Including a sufficient number of athletes to get strong statistical power
- Minimizing any confounding effects from extraneous factors that are not part of the study
- Precisely measuring performance and physiological variables that the supplement may affect
- Implementing proper training protocols to accurately reveal the supplement's utility

Some supplements display scientific references on the label to substantiate use of that product. While this practice can be helpful, some deception can take place, as research findings are often taken out of context.

In terms of ergogenicity, many supplements get a failing grade by rigorous scientific standards. Many supplements have failed to enhance performance when consumed at the manufacturer's recommended dosages. However, it is quite common to see athletes consume nutrition supplements at doses that far exceed the recommended range. Anecdotally, testimonials in several magazine articles, advertisements, and interviews with well-known athletes have suggested some of these supplements to be ergogenic when taken at supraphysiological doses. However, few scientific studies have examined supplement doses in that high range, so it is unclear if the statements have any merit. Using consistency as a standard, only a few supplements have repeatedly proven to be advantageous.

Physiological Relevance of Supplement Use

The key questions to ask when appraising potential supplements for use are: What is the supplement's physiological relevance and what is the supplement supposed to do? The answers to these questions may require some background knowledge of physiology, which is provided in subsequent chapters in this book. The supplement in question must have some involvement in the processes affecting acute and chronic performance and training adaptations. If the supplement appears to have no benefit on the surface, then that supplement is likely not worthy of use physiologically or economically.

Supplement Use Among Athletes

Sport-supplement use in athletes has increased in popularity over the years. Historically, athletic departments were allowed to distribute supplements to student-athletes.

However, that practice is no longer tolerated, as controversies involving some supplements (e.g., creatine, prohormones, and ephedra) have led to imposed limitations on supplement distribution by the athletic department. Nevertheless, student-athletes still have unlimited access to sport supplements provided they are purchased outside of the school setting. One study by Burns and colleagues showed that out of eight NCAA I universities, 80 percent of the 228 athletes surveyed reported using one supplement and 58 percent reported using at least two sports supplements as part of their training. Most studies have shown that, on average, more than 50 percent of athletes consume nutrition supplements, and the higher the level of competition, the greater the prevalence of supplement use (i.e., elite athletes are the most frequent consumers). Among the supplements consumed, vitamin/minerals, calorie-replacement drinks, proteins/amino acids, and creatine are the most popular.

Although elite athletes may be the predominant supplement consumers, a trickle-down effect exists, and young athletes are supplementing more now than ever before. High school and middle school student-athletes are becoming aware of the popularity of sports supplements through friends, magazines, and the media (e.g., reports of famous athletes using supplements). Great pressure to win from coaches, parents, and friends, coupled with the fact that some athletes are now turning professional out of high school, may cause young athletes to view supplement use as a means to achieving greater success. In fact, a 2001 study by Metzl and colleagues looked at creatine use in sixth through twelfth grades and found that approximately 6 percent of students had taken creatine. The highest rate was observed in twelfth graders (44 percent), and gymnastics, hockey, wrestling, football, lacrosse, and weight training were the sports and activities that saw the highest incidence of creatine use. When the scientists investigated potential reasons for creatine use among these populations, the most common responses were enhanced performance, appearance, speed, and endurance.

Other popular supplements among high school athletes are multivitamins and minerals, amino acid and protein, weight gainers, HMB, sport drinks, and prohormones (although prohormones have been banned from over-the-counter sales). A 2004 study by Bartee and colleagues revealed the following trends among 1,737 ninth through twelfth graders surveyed:

- Boys had a 87 percent greater chance of using supplements than girls
- Twelfth graders were 64 percent more likely to supplement than ninth graders
- Students who participated in two or more sports were most likely to supplement
- Athletes with a favorable outlook on supplement use had a 13 times greater likelihood of consuming supplements
- Athletes with supportive parents or guardians were more likely to use supplements

Interestingly, a study by Massad and colleagues (1995) showed that supplement use declined when high school athletes were educated properly about supplements.

Sources of Supplement Knowledge Among Athletes

Where athletes get their information on sports supplements is very important. Due to the mass marketing of supplements and exaggerated claims on labels and in advertisements, it is very easy for athletes to be fed misinformation. Virtually every supplement advertisement claims some ergogenic element that enhances performance, which leaves the athlete in a tempting situation. You should take an active role in leading your athletes to credible sources on sports supplements. In Division I athletics, athletic trainers and strength and conditioning coaches are often sought out for supplement information. However, other reports show that friends, teammates, and magazines are often prime sources of supplement information, which means that the chances of athletes receiving misinformation are very likely. Properly educating athletes is essential.

Athletes' Age and Level of Training

At what age should athletes begin taking nutrition supplements? The answer to this question is not simple, as many young athletes become fascinated with the supplement industry and some experiment with supplements at an early age, especially since some of their professional athlete role models are spokespersons for various supplements. Many young athletes feel compelled to start supplementing early to get ahead of the competition. Athletes turning pro out of high school do very little to curtail this phenomenon. The basic premise is that if it helps, then the young athlete will try it. But, should this trend be the norm or the exception?

The key element is the level of maturity and training experience of the young athlete. Teenagers' bodies are still in the developmental stage. Growth spurts take place at periodic phases and hormonal changes are evident, meaning that the possibility of training adaptations is still very large and normal dietary intake supplies adequate amounts of nutrients to sustain training at this level. Perhaps a multivitamin or some additional carbohydrates and protein may be useful at this stage, but other supplements do not appear necessary in most cases. Historically, supplement use has been most effective when used to overcome training plateaus. That is, many individuals (especially resistance-trained athletes such as strength competitors, bodybuilders, Olympic weight lifters, and power lifters) establish a firm training base during the first few years of training and later use supplements when progression becomes more difficult. With this model in mind, it makes sense for young athletes to train smart and eat right initially, develop a firm conditioning base, and then supplement in later years (i.e., late teens to early twenties). Using this technique, supplements may be used in a more efficient manner to surpass plateaus when gains become somewhat more difficult to obtain.

A prime example of establishing a training base before supplementing is evident in a common criticism of several sport-supplement studies. Some research studies have been criticized for using previously untrained individuals as subjects due to the high learning curve associated with the initial training phase. It is a fact that adaptations of the nervous system predominate early in training, and untrained subjects respond favorably regardless of the training program. Testing a supplement or even a training program at this point is extremely difficult because any potential differentiating effects may be overshadowed by the learning curve. For example, some creatine-supplementation studies have shown no ergogenic benefits in untrained subjects (although some studies have shown benefits). But why use a known ergogenic at a time when gains should be prevalent anyway? These studies lack a practical application, but an analogy can be made to young athletes. As long as gains are being made through training alone, sports supplements may not be necessary until the rate of progression has slowed significantly.

An exception to this model may be caused by the level of competition encountered by the athlete. Young, elite athletes competing in sports in which peak performance and success may be attained at a young age (e.g., gymnastics) may benefit from the use of some supplements. Competing at that elite level may supersede typical supplementation guidelines.

Bioavailability—Does the Supplement Get to Where It Needs to Be?

Bioavailability refers to how much of a consumed supplement actually reaches the target site. The supplement needs to end up in its proper location for the desired effects to occur. Bioavailability is determined by the nature and formulation of the supplement. For example, L-carnitine has been used as a "fat burner" because of its role as a transporter of fatty acids in the muscle's mitochondria (i.e., the site of aerobic energy metabolism within the cell). Although supplementation studies have shown a higher level of L-carnitine in the blood, no elevation in L-carnitine concentration within the muscle has been documented. These results show that supplemental L-carnitine does not reach the target area, which casts doubt on the effectiveness of its use in this context. In fact, some studies have shown no affect on body composition with L-carnitine supplementation.

Supplement Patterns

The pattern of supplementation refers to the method by which the supplement is taken. In other words, is it more effective to take a constant dose of a supplement regularly over a long period of time or to "cycle" a supplement based on the training phase? The answer depends on the supplement in question. Supplements used to correct a deficiency are most often taken at consistent doses over a period of time. Supplementing with 400 international units (IU) of vitamin E per day over the course of a year is a common example. Taking more than the needed amount provides no further benefit. Therefore, a constant dose is sufficient to maintain optimal levels of intake.

Considering that the majority of benefits that occur with "ergogenic" supplements take place during the initial phase of supplementation, some authorities have suggested that cycling supplements may be more effective for getting a more substantial, long-term effect. Cycling refers to a pattern of use in which the athlete takes the supplement for a period of time (usually six to 12 weeks), and then reduces the dose over time until use of the supplement is terminated. After a period of training without the supplement, the athlete will then initiate another cycle further into the training period. The rationale behind cycling is to increase performance during supplementation, maintain as much of the performance gain as possible without supplement use (i.e., a residual effect), and begin a new supplementation cycle at a higher training base than the previous cycle. A supplement with which cycling may be useful is creatine. Figure 1-4 presents a theoretical application of cycling of the supplement creatine.

Label Accuracy

An accurately labeled supplement is important to the athlete. Stated simply, the supplement should be composed of what is stated on the label. Although the United States Food and Drug Administration set standards for the testing, promotion, and advertising of prescription drugs, sports supplements are less tightly controlled. The impact of a mislabeled supplement on the athlete could be as simple as a supplement that is less effective, or it could mean the possibility of a failed drug test if the supplement is contaminated with a banned substance such as a prohormone or anabolic steroid.

Dose Response and Toxicity

A dose-response relationship indicates how much of an effect is obtained from the supplement at various levels of consumption. For most supplements that correct a deficiency in athletes, the amount of supplement taken may be more than the recommended daily allowance (RDA). Therefore, any more will be of no additional benefit. Activity level, as well as other circumstances, increases the nutrient requirements. Taking more than what is necessary provides no further advantage to an athlete. For some ergogenic supplements that are pharmaceutical in nature, a more sufficient response may be present with gradually increasing doses. Nevertheless, a

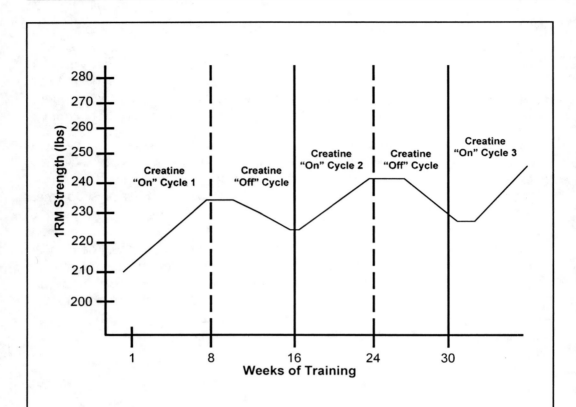

In this model, creatine supplementation corresponds to strength phases. Cycle 1 increases the athlete's one-repetition maximum (1 RM) by approximately 25 pounds. During a subsequent eight-week reduced intake/off phase, 1-RM strength is maintained to a higher degree than that of the baseline level established before cycle 1. This additional retainment is known as a "residual" effect from the previous supplement cycle. A second creatine cycle is used and the athlete again increases 1-RM strength to a greater degree than in the previous cycle. In this model, the goals are to optimize residual strength (i.e., strength independent of the supplement), begin a new strength phase at a higher baseline level, and finish the phase with a greater 1 RM than the previous phase.

Figure 1-4. Theoretical model for creatine cycling

common—and erroneous—thought is that if "X" amount of a supplement works, than increasing the dose substantially to "Y" will have a greater effect. The truth is that athletes taking supraphysiological doses of supplements over an extended period of time run the risk of toxicity, a negative health manifestation due to consumption of too large a dose of supplements.

The "Placebo" Effect

A psychological component exists with supplementation. In some instances, the athlete thinks the supplement will enhance performance and he subsequently trains harder. Improvement in performance may occur, but this improvement is most likely due to the athlete's enhanced training initiative and not to the supplement itself. The improvement occurs as a result of what is called the "placebo" effect. A placebo is a fake (in the sense that it has no physiological value) pill or powder given to subjects or patients in studies as a control to investigate the effects of another drug or supplement. Many times an athlete's improved performance has been falsely attributed to a particular supplement when in fact the athlete was training more intensely under the assumption that the supplement was working. The placebo effects is yet another reason why it is important for you to base your decisions on scientifically controlled studies rather than anecdotal information.

Responders vs. Nonresponders

Many studies that have shown the ergogenic properties of supplements do not have 100 percent of the subjects showing the same rate of improvement. In some cases, some subjects do not improve at all. A "responder" is an athlete who achieves a high level of performance enhancement from supplementation. A "nonresponder," therefore, is someone who receives very little, if any, benefit. Scientists have tried to identify reasons why some individuals have no response when the majority of subjects/athletes in a study experience improvements. Although the reason is not clear, individual physiological differences (e.g., muscle-fiber composition) appear evident.

Ethics

Ethics may be defined as the moral principles by which an individual or sport association self-governs. The use of sports supplements raises a few ethical questions. One "purist" school of thought is that an athlete should make the best of his training and dietary food intake, and limit or avoid supplement intake. Another school of thought is to be the best that is humanly possible, which entails supplementing to maximize performance during training and competition. Whether an athlete chooses to supplement depends on the his values and the legality of the supplement(s) in question. Macronutrients, vitamins and minerals, and many other supplements are legal, and these substances are found in abundance in the human body and in the typical diet. An athlete's choice to supplement with these compounds raises very few questions pertaining to ethical values. However, pharmacological agents are banned substances in most competitions and some are illegal to possess without a prescription for medical purposes. The use of these substances is unethical, though many athletes use them to gain a competitive advantage. A typical response from an athlete who has been caught using these substances is, "I had to because most of the competition is using them as well." This response raises a potentially interesting issue: Is it cheating if most athletes are doing the same thing? While this question may not be easily answered in the minds of some individuals, drug use is still illegal, and you must advise your athletes to do what is right.

2

Carbohydrates

Carbohydrates, which are categorized as monosaccharides, disaccharides, and oligosaccharides/polysaccharides, are macromolecules consisting of carbon, hydrogen, and oxygen atoms. *Monosaccharides* are basic carbohydrate units that consist of glucose, fructose, and galactose. Although monosaccharides are the simplest form of carbohydrates, only glucose can be used by muscles for energy. Therefore, fructose and galactose must be converted to glucose in the liver prior to use. Disaccharides consist of two monosaccharides. Both di- and monosaccharides are considered simple sugars based on their structures and ease of breakdown. *Disaccharides* include sucrose (glucose-plus-fructose), lactose (glucose-plus-galactose), and maltose (glucose-plus-glucose). Sucrose is the most commonly consumed disaccharide in the United States, as it is contained in table sugar and honey. Lactose is mostly found in milk, and maltose is found in breakfast cereals. *Oligosaccharides* consist of three to nine monosaccharides, while *polysaccharides* consist of more than 10 monosaccharides.

Polysaccharides include starch, glycogen, and fiber. Starch is a complex carbohydrate found in abundance in grain products (e.g., pasta, rice, cereal, and bread) and corn. Glycogen is the storage form of carbohydrates in humans and is very important for rapid use of glucose during high-intensity exercise. Most glycogen is stored in skeletal muscle (300 to 500 grams). However, some glycogen (75 to 100 grams) is stored in the liver, which is crucial to increasing blood-sugar levels during exercise. Fiber (both soluble and insoluble) is indigestible, so the intake of fiber enhances the excretion of fats and other substances that can have a negative impact on health. Diets high in fiber (25 to 35 grams per day) have been shown to reduce hunger as well as the risk of gastrointestinal disease, cardiovascular disease, and various forms of cancer. Excellent food sources of fiber include fruits, vegetables, legumes, and grain products.

Functions of Carbohydrates

Carbohydrates perform many functions critical to optimal performance and athletic success (Figure 2-1). A critical function of carbohydrates is to act as a source of energy for the human body. Adenosine triphosphate (ATP) is used for energy in the human body and is liberated via three basic energy systems (two anaerobic and one aerobic). The major means by which carbohydrates provide energy is through a process called *glycolysis*, which involves the breaking down of glucose for energy. Glucose is obtained via transport into the cell from the blood (i.e., via an increase in blood sugar) or through a process called *glycogenolysis*, which is the breaking down of glycogen from either the muscle or liver stores. Glycogenolysis is regulated by enzymes (under hormonal control) and this process is critical to energy production during high-intensity exercise and competition.

- Provide energy for optimal exercise performance

- Provide energy for the central nervous system

- Maintain cell structure and integrity

- Enhance function of the immune system

- Act as a structural component of genetic material (DNA and RNA)

- Regulate lipid metabolism, amino-acid metabolism, and protein synthesis and breakdown by stimulating the secretion of the anabolic hormone *insulin*

- Increase thermogenesis

Figure 2-1. Functions of carbohydrates

The rate of glycogen depletion is related to exercise intensity, and muscle glycogen is the predominant source of glucose during moderate-to-high intensity exercise of sufficient duration. Lactic acid, which is formed during anaerobic glycolysis, is a major factor leading to muscular fatigue. Lactic acid is shuttled from the muscles to the blood, where it may be used for energy, converted to glucose, or converted into liver glycogen. Lactic-acid production during exercise rises exponentially after a threshold intensity is reached of approximately 55 to 60 percent of maximal oxygen consumption in lesser-trained athletes and 70 to 80 percent in trained athletes.

Carbohydrate Intake

Carbohydrate intake should make up a large component of an athlete's diet. The total amount of carbohydrates consumed on a daily basis (as well as daily caloric intake) depends upon the athlete's size, level of conditioning, and activity level. It is recommended that an athlete consume approximately 55 to 65 percent of his calories from carbohydrates. The majority of carbohydrates should be complex in nature with less than 10 percent derived from simple carbohydrates. Complex carbohydrates should be derived mostly from meals, whereas simple carbohydrates can be derived from meals and through supplements. A common intake is approximately 6 grams of carbohydrate (CHO) per kilogram of body mass each day. The timing of carbohydrate intake is also of great importance. Critical carbohydrate-intake times include days before training or competition, hours before training or competition, during training or competition, and after training or competition.

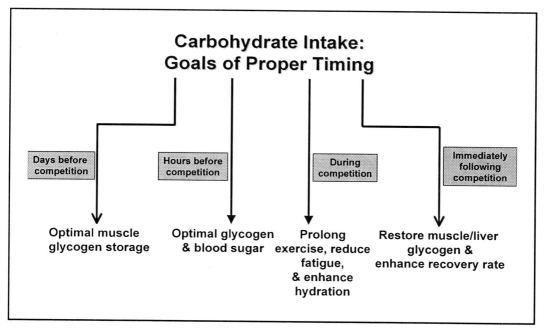

Figure 2-2. Goals of carbohydrate intake at various times

Glycemic Index

The glycemic index is a reference system (based on a standardized amount of glucose) pertaining to the elevation in blood sugar and insulin in response to dietary food and beverage consumption. The glycemic index has important ramifications for the time of food consumption prior to, and/or during, exercise, as well as for appetite control. The index consists of averaged values based on high-, moderate-, and low-index foods. For example, glucose has an index value of 100. This value indicates that a rapid increase in blood glucose will occur following glucose consumption. Foods with a high glycemic index (greater than 70) result in rapid elevations in blood sugar. Some examples of high-glycemic foods include pancakes, baked potatoes, pretzels, and some cereals. Moderate-glycemic foods (56 to 70) increase blood sugar at a slower rate than high-index foods and beverages. Some examples of moderate-glycemic foods include doughnuts, muffins, candy bars, and rice. Low-glycemic foods (less than 55) raise blood-sugar levels more slowly than moderate- and high-index foods. Some examples include legumes, some fruits and vegetables, and yogurt. Although the use of the glycemic index may be controversial at times—because some foods high in complex carbohydrates have high indices and some simple sugars are low on the index, in addition to the fact these numbers may change based on other foods consumed simultaneously and individual differences—it does give coaches and athletes an indication of the response time for certain foods.

A newer concept that may have greater application to the change in blood-sugar levels is the glycemic load. The *glycemic load* is based on the total carbohydrate content of a serving of food instead of on a standardized glucose reference point. The glycemic load equals the glycemic index multiplied by the carbohydrate content. As with the glycemic index, the glycemic load has low (less than 10), medium (11 to 19), and high (greater than 20) classifications. Although little research has been done in this area, some experts have suggested that athletes should consume lower glycemic index or load foods prior to exercise and consume higher glycemic index or load foods during and following exercise or competition to have quick elevations in blood sugar, delay fatigue, and increase the rate of recovery.

Types of Carbohydrate Supplements

Carbohydrate supplements typically are sports drinks and sports nutrition bars, gels, tablets/capsules, and powders (for mixture). Although carbohydrates are readily available in foods and beverages, supplements have an advantage because they are rapidly broken down and used for energy. Other advantages to supplements are that they are easy to transport and consume, a large quantity of carbohydrates can be consumed in a short period of time before, during, and after competition, and supplement beverages quench thirst and can be used for rehydrating the athlete during long competitions in hot, humid weather. Many sport drinks contain approximately 6 to 8 percent of their volume as carbohydrates in the form of glucose, fructose, sucrose, and glucose polymers. Besides replenishing glucose and glycogen, the quantity of carbohydrates in a sport drink is important for optimizing gastric emptying. Too many

High Glycemic Index Foods (greater than 70)

Food	GI	GL
Pancakes	102	22
Pretzels	83	16
Rice Krispies®	82	22
Corn Flakes®	81	21
Jelly beans	78	22
Gatorade®	78	12
Waffles	76	10
French fries	75	22
Mashed potatoes	74	15
Cheerios®	74	15
Bagels	72	25
Pop Tarts®	70	24
Life Savers®	70	21
White bread	70	10

Moderate Glycemic Index Foods (56–70)

Food	GI	GL
Coca-Cola®	58	15
Raisin Bran®	61	12
Snickers® bar	68	23
Mars® bar	65	26
Cranberry juice cocktail	68	24
Couscous	65	23
White rice	64	23
Instant white rice	69	29
Ice cream	61	8
Power Bar® (chocolate)	56	24

Low Glycemic Index Foods (less than 56)

Food	GI	GL	Food	GI	GL
Milk (with fat)	27	3	Strawberries	40	1
Chocolate milk	43	12	Baked Beans	48	7
Skim milk	27	4	Butter Beans	36	7
Juices (apple, orange, tomato, carrot, grapefruit, pineapple)	37–50	10–13	Kidney Beans	23	6
			Linguine	52	23
			Macaroni	47	23
Wheat bread	53	11	Fettucine	40	18
All-Bran® cereal	38	9	Pure Protein Bars	22-43	2-6
Soy milk	32	7	Peanuts	14	1
Apples	38	6	Tomato Soup	38	6
Bananas	52	12	Green Peas	48	3
Grapes	46	8	Carrots	47	3
Oranges	42	5	Honey	55	10
Peaches	42	5	Yogurt	36	3
Pears	38	4			

*Adapted from Foster-Powell et al. (2002)

Figure 2-3. Glycemic index (GI) and glycemic load (GL) values for selected foods

carbohydrates in a beverage can impede fluid absorption (e.g., greater than 6 percent of total volume) and limit rehydration. In addition, sport drinks have electrolytes (sodium and potassium), which also are important for rehydration. Many carbohydrate supplements taste good, and thereby increase the likelihood that the athlete will consume adequate amounts. Prime supplemental periods include during and immediately after exercise/competition. It is more difficult to consume a meal during these times, so drinks or bars are popular choices. An athlete may not be hungry initially after a competition or training session, and consuming a sport drink or bar is important when hunger is not present (although greater thirst will be present). When coaching endurance-oriented events or long-duration sports, it is important to stress carbohydrate supplementation and have supplements (drinks) available for the athletes to consume during and after competition. The athletic training (or medical) staff plays a prominent role in monitoring the athletes' hydration status, especially during exercise or competition in hot, humid environments.

Carbohydrate Intake Prior to Exercise

Adequate carbohydrate intake on the days leading up to competition is important for maximizing muscle-glycogen stores. Intake may be in the form of meals that are high in complex carbohydrates. Proper intake ensures that muscle glycogen is restored from previous workouts, especially if the athlete tapers prior to the competition (i.e., performs a short period of low-volume, low-intensity, and low-frequency workouts prior to major competition).

Another common nutritional practice is carbohydrate loading. Carbohydrate loading involves depletion of glycogen stores, consumption of large amounts of carbohydrates, and subsequent glycogen replenishment. However, the goal of *carbohydrate loading* is to overcompensate for glycogen storage. That is, the athlete may be able to store more muscle glycogen than normal based on this pattern of depletion-repletion. For example, an athlete will engage in a very demanding exercise session that results in significant glycogen depletion. The athlete then consumes a low-carbohydrate diet over a three-day period. Another exhausting exercise session is then performed. However, following this session, the athlete consumes a high-carbohydrate diet for the next three days. This process is known as a "classical model of supercompensation" and has been shown to elevate muscle-glycogen levels beyond those of normal training and diet. However, some negative side effects have been seen with this model (e.g., gastric distress, hypoglycemia, poor performance during the low-carbohydrate phase, mood swings), which has led scientists to develop other more accommodating ways of increasing glycogen storage beyond normal. For example, tapering during training accommodated by high levels of carbohydrate intake has also been shown to increase muscle-glycogen levels comparable to those seen with the classic model. The newer system is less stressful to the athlete and may be easier to incorporate into training/competition cycles.

Research has shown that carbohydrate loading or high-carbohydrate diets (e.g., 500 to 650 grams per day) can increase muscle- and liver-glycogen content to as much as 1.8 times that of a normal diet in men and women (especially when 8 to 10.5 grams of carbohydrates per kilogram of body mass per day were consumed over three days). The higher glycogen content in muscle appears to last approximately three days following loading, so exercise or competition performed during this time could potentially be enhanced. However, performance has not always been shown to improve. The intensity and duration of exercise are important considerations. No benefit appears to be associated with carbohydrate loading before short-term, high-intensity activities (e.g., sprinting, weight training). Only some studies have shown performance improvement during exercise sessions lasting one hour or less, but more substantial improvements have been seen with exercise sessions lasting longer than 90 minutes. Overall, high-carbohydrate diets have been estimated to improve endurance by approximately 20 percent and the performance of fixed-distance activities by 2 to 3 percent.

Although carbohydrate loading may appear to offer some benefits for endurance events (e.g., marathons, triathlons), it does not appear that carbohydrate loading is feasible for sports involving multiple competitions/practices in a short period of time. These types of competition or game schedules require optimal performance several times each week. Therefore, the athlete cannot afford (and does not have time) to deplete glycogen levels and then supercompensate or he runs the risk of suboptimal practice, a greater risk of stomach distress, rapid changes in body weight (as water is also stored as glycogen is stored), hypoglycemia (i.e., low blood sugar), reduced cognitive function, and poor performance. Some studies have shown performance enhancement in these sports when athletes have higher levels of glycogen. Therefore, it is recommended that these athletes consume a diet high in carbohydrates (55 to 65 percent of caloric intake, or 500 to 650 grams per day) without periods of depletion/repletion.

The consumption of a substantial amount of carbohydrates within four hours of an endurance training/competition is also important. High carbohydrate intake during this time frame increases blood-sugar levels and slightly increases glycogen content, both of which can enhance endurance performance during long events. Williams (1998) recommended the following precompetition carbohydrate-intake strategy:

- Four hours precompetition: 4 grams per kilogram of body mass
- One hour precompetition: 1 gram per kilogram of body mass
- 10 minutes precompetition: 0.5 grams per kilogram of body mass

Supplementation During Exercise

Carbohydrate supplementation during endurance events of at least moderate intensity or during long competitions lasting at least 90 minutes appears to positively affect sports performance. Carbohydrate supplementation during prolonged exercise is thought to maintain blood-sugar levels, spare muscle and liver glycogen, and promote glycogen synthesis (i.e., during rest periods between intermittent bouts or periods of low-intensity activity), which delays the onset of fatigue. In addition, the human body tends to rely more on consumed carbohydrates during strenuous exercise in an attempt to preserve bodily stores. Carbohydrates consumed through supplementation can only be used at a rate of approximately 1.0 to 1.2 grams per minute. Therefore, it has been recommended that athletes consume approximately 30 to 70 grams of carbohydrates per hour during long-term exercise, depending on the intensity of the exercise, the size of the athlete, the type of carbohydrates consumed, and the conditioning level of the athlete. The carbohydrates can be consumed all at once or at regular fixed intervals (e.g., every 15 minutes). Any additional carbohydrate intake beyond this level will not increase use to a greater extent or improve performance, but may lead to other side effects such as stomach distress. The carbohydrates selected should consist mostly of glucose, sucrose, and maltose, as other sugars (e.g., fructose, galactose) take longer to metabolize.

Postworkout Supplementation

Carbohydrate intake following a competition is critical to optimizing recovery. This concept becomes increasingly important if another competition is scheduled within days of the one just completed. The athlete's postgame meal or supplementation is the first step in the preparation for the next competition or practice session and marks the beginning of the recovery period. Strategies to optimize recovery between sessions or competitions are critical to you and your athletes in preparation for the next event.

The restoration of muscle and liver glycogen is important in the initial recovery period. The process of glycogen repletion or synthesis involves many factors (e.g., action of certain hormones, getting glucose into the muscle cells, blood flow), but one critical factor is the amount of carbohydrate present in supplement or meal form. A key enzyme in promoting glycogen storage is *glycogen synthase* and its activity is very high following training, especially when blood-sugar levels are high. Trained individuals have a higher activity of glycogen synthase and higher levels of resting muscle-glycogen content. Glycogen repletion is biphasic, with a rapid early phase during the first 24 hours and a slower phase potentially lasting a few days. The following steps should be taken by the athlete for optimal glycogen repletion:

- The athlete should obtain a high-glycemic carbohydrate supplement as soon as possible following the event (liquid or solid, although liquids are important for rehydration and the athlete may not be hungry at this point in time).

- The supplement should consist of mostly glucose for rapid uptake, but some studies show that added amino acids may also help. If protein is added, a 3:1 ratio of carbohydrate to protein should be used.

- For rapid glycogen repletion, the athlete should consume 1.5 grams of carbohydrates per kilogram of body mass within 30 minutes. This intake should be repeated every two hours for four to six hours.

- For slower repletion, the athlete should consume 8 to 10 grams per kilogram of body mass over a 24-hour period.

Coaching Points

- Athletes should consume approximately 55 to 65 percent of calories from carbohydrates (less than 10 percent from simple sugars), which is equivalent to approximately six grams of carbohydrate per kilogram of body mass per day, mostly from low-glycemic foods.

- Critical carbohydrate-intake times include days before training or competition, hours before training or competition, during training and competition, and after training or competition.

- A suggested strategy for precompetition carbohydrate intake entails consuming four grams per kilogram of body mass four hours precompetition, 1 gram per kilogram of body mass one hour precompetition and 0.5 grams per kilogram of body mass 10 minutes precompetition.

- It is recommended that athletes consume approximately 30 to 70 grams of carbohydrates per hour during long-term exercise (at 15-minute intervals), depending on the intensity of the exercise, the size of the athlete, the type of carbohydrates consumed, and the conditioning level of the athlete.

- For rapid glycogen repletion after competition/training, the athlete should consume 1.5 grams of carbohydrate per kilogram of body mass within 30 minutes and repeat this intake every two hours for four to six hours.

- For slower repletion following competition, the athlete should 8 to 10 grams per kilogram of body mass over a 24-hour period.

3

Protein and Amino Acids

Protein is a large macronutrient made up of building blocks called *amino acids*. A protein consists of a specifically sequenced chain of more than 100 amino acids linked together. Of the 20 amino acids that have been identified, nine are "essential" and 11 are "nonessential." *Nonessential* amino acids can be produced within the body, whereas *essential* amino acids must be obtained through the diet. The structure of a protein dictates its function and is dependent upon the biochemical interaction of amino acids within the chain. More than 10,000 proteins have been identified, each with specific functions. Of primary importance to you and your athletes

Essential	Nonessential
Leucine	Alanine
Isoleucine	Arginine
Valine	Asparagine
Histidine	Aspartic acid
Methionine	Cysteine
Phenylalanine	Glutamic acid
Threonine	Glutamine
Tryptophan	Glycine
Lysine	Proline
	Serine
	Tyrosine

Note: Italics indicate branched-chain amino acids

Figure 3-1. Essential and nonessential amino acids

among the many functions of proteins and amino acids are the roles they play in increasing muscle size, strength, power, and endurance, and in recovery between workouts and games/competitions.

Enzymes—Proteins act as enzymes that catalyze nearly all reactions in the human body.

Transport and Storage—Proteins are involved in transporting molecules (e.g., hormones, oxygen) in the blood and storing molecules within the cells. In addition, proteins located within the cell membrane regulate what goes in and out of the cell (and how much).

Hormones and Receptors—Proteins act as hormones in the body. Some important protein hormones involved in increasing muscle size and strength are insulin, insulin-like growth factor-1, and human growth hormone. Proteins act as receptors and are necessary to mediate the hormonal response. In addition, some amino acids are thought to stimulate a hormonal response.

Immune System Support—Many immune cells are proteins that help the body fight disease and improve recovery ability.

Nerve Transmission—Some amino acids form neurotransmitters, which are necessary for proper nerve function.

Mechanical Support—Certain proteins (e.g., collagen) are essential to maintaining the strength of tendons, ligaments, bones, skin, organs, etc.

Muscle Function—Proteins form the contractile unit that enables muscles to contract and produce force. In addition, structural proteins are necessary to stabilize these proteins as well as the muscle itself.

Energy—Certain amino acids (e.g., alanine, leucine) may be used for energy during times of starvation or strenuous endurance exercise.

Acid-Base Balance—Proteins can buffer acids to preserve blood and muscle pH.

Figure 3-2. Basic functions of proteins and amino acids

Growth and Recovery

Muscle growth and recovery necessitate that the amount of protein synthesized be greater than the amount broken down. A reduction in breakdown and/or an increase in synthesis results in a positive net protein balance, which is what the athlete seeks through proper training, diet, and supplementation. Protein synthesis is elevated from three to 48 hours following a weight-training workout. In fact, both breakdown and synthesis are greater after a workout. However, the rate of synthesis is far greater than breakdown within 48 hours following exercise, leaving the athlete with a positive protein balance. Prolonged periods of positive protein balance lead to muscle growth and recovery, and potential increases in strength and power. Factors such as the metabolic and mechanical stress from lifting weights (and the training program used), the muscles' hydration status, and the acute anabolic hormonal response (e.g., testosterone, growth hormone, insulin-like growth factor-1) contribute to and enhance protein synthesis, muscle growth, and recovery.

Sources of Protein

Food sources consisting of protein may be classified as *complete* or *incomplete*. Complete sources of protein contain all of the essential amino acids in adequate quantities and include meat, poultry, fish, dairy products, and soy protein. Incomplete proteins lack one or more essential amino acids and include vegetables, grains, and nuts. Complete proteins tend to be more efficient (i.e., better absorption and utilization). Therefore, complete sources of protein should be included in every athlete's diet.

Types of Protein Supplements

Proteins differ based on their source, amino-acid composition, and the method of processing or isolation. Proteins from animal sources are of the highest quality based on rating scales (e.g., protein-efficiency ratio, biological value, net protein utilization, and protein digestibility–corrected amino acid score). Protein supplements also contain other mixtures of protein from whey, casein, soy, and bovine colostrum.

Whey proteins are purified and separated from cow's milk following the manufacturing of cheese. They contain high levels of essential and branched-chain amino acids (BCAA)—especially leucine—and are easy to digest. Whey protein contains an ample supply of the amino acid cysteine, which plays a role in enhancing the immune system. The major forms of whey are powder, concentrate, and isolates. The isolates are the purest form of protein, while the concentrates contain more biologically active components and contain little to no fat, lactose, or cholesterol. In addition, the composition of whey protein is similar to that of skeletal muscle (i.e., the amino-acid concentrations are in a similar proportion).

Casein makes up the majority (approximately 70 to 80 percent) of bovine milk protein (40 percent in humans), whereas whey constitutes about 20 percent. Casein, which is the curd that forms when milk sours, also contains a large proportion of essential amino acids. Because casein is not dissolvable in water, caseinates (salts of casein that are water-soluble) are typically found in protein supplements (e.g., calcium and sodium caseinates).

Soy protein, the most widely used vegetable protein, is complete, with all essential amino acids. Soy is high in branched-chain amino acids and scores very highly in protein-rating scales.

Bovine colostrum is the premilk fluid produced by the mother's mammary glands during the first 72 hours after birth. Colostrum provides life-supporting immune and growth factors that stimulate the amount of proteins synthesized.

Comparisons have been made between the various protein sources and their effects on performance enhancement. Most studies used whey and bovine colostrum because whey can be used as an effective placebo (i.e., it tastes and looks similar to colostrum). The results of these studies demonstrate strengths and weaknesses for each protein source, although it is difficult to draw firm conclusions because some studies have contradicted others (Figure 3-3). Colostrum supplementation may elevate insulin-like growth factor-1 (IGF-1, a potent anabolic hormone for muscle growth) concentrations in the blood and lean body mass more than whey protein, although other studies do not support these findings. The possibility of an elevation in lean body mass may suggest that athletes such as body builders (i.e., those who strive to increase muscle size) may benefit slightly from colostrum supplementation.

Colostrum has not been shown to enhance muscular strength or endurance any more than whey protein. However, colostrum may improve performance of a second bout of exercise following the first bout, thereby suggesting enhanced recovery between exercise sessions. Digestion of whey protein leads to a quick appearance of amino acids in the blood, whereas casein protein is absorbed more slowly and results in a slow increase in blood amino acids. Whey also leads to a greater rate of protein synthesis than casein, possibly due to the higher proportion of leucine found in whey proteins. Leucine is a branched-chain amino acid that can increase protein synthesis. Soy protein contains a substantial amount of antioxidants and reduces inflammation following resistance exercise and protein breakdown, which may enhance recovery to a greater extent than whey or casein proteins.

It is understandably difficult for a coach to decide what source of protein may provide the most benefits to his athletes It appears that a combination of protein sources may be most advantageous. Many supplements on the market do contain proteins from more than one source. Studies have shown that 20 to 60 grams each day of protein from whey, casein, soy, and bovine colostrum sources may be effective for enhancing some facets of performance.

Reference	Supplement	Protocol	Results
Antonio et al. (2001)	BC or whey 20 g/day	8 weeks of weight and aerobic training	BC greater ↑ in LBM; no difference in performance
Brinkworth et al. (2004)	BC or whey 60 g/day	8 weeks of weight training for the biceps	BC greater ↑ in CSA; no difference in strength
Buckley et al. (2003)	BC or whey 60 g/day	8 weeks of weight and plyometric training	BC greater ↑ in VJ and cycling power; no difference in strength
Buckley et al. (2002)	BC or whey 60 g/day	8 weeks of running	BC 5.2% greater ↑ in endurance in a second bout 20 minutes after the first bout
Hofman et al. (2002)	BC or whey 60 g/day	8 weeks of anaerobic training	BC greater ↑ in sprint time; no difference in body composition or endurance
Brinkworth et al. (2002)	BC or whey 60 g/day	9 weeks of training for competitive rowing	BC greater ↑ in buffer capacity; no difference in performance
Coombes et al. (2002)	BC 20 g/day + whey 40 g/day; BC 60 g/day; or whey 60 g/day	8 weeks of cycle training	20 and 60 g BC small ↑ in cycle time trial performance
Laskowski & Antosiewicz (2003)	Soy 0.5 g/kg of body mass/day vs. control	4 weeks of judo training	Soy greater ↑ in $\dot{V}O_2$ max and anaerobic power

Note: g = gram; kg = kilogram; ↑ = increase; BC = bovine colostrum; LBM = lean body mass; CSA = muscle cross-sectional area; VJ = vertical jump

Figure 3-3. Comparison of whey, soy, casein, and colostrum protein sources on athletic performance

Protein Supplementation Guidelines and Timing

Athletes require higher protein intake than the recommended daily allowance (RDA) value, and intake will depend upon factors such as the intensity, volume, and frequency of training. Strength and power athletes should consume approximately 1.7 to 2.2 grams per kilogram of body mass of protein per day (or at least double the RDA). The average recommendation for a strength and power athlete is 1.8 grams per kilogram of body mass, or approximately 180 grams per day for the 100-kilogram (220-pound) athlete. Supplementation is recommended if the athlete does not consume an adequate amount from the diet. Protein supplements contain various amounts of

Supplement	Kilocalories	Protein (grams)	Carbohydrate (grams)	Fat (grams)
EAS Myo Pro Whey	115	21	3	2
Labrada V-60 Protein	~155	30	6	1
AST VP2 Whey Protein Isolate	100	24	1	<0.5
Optimum Nutrition 100% Whey Protein	110	22	2	1.5
Optimum Nutrition Pro Complex	260	55	3	3
Champion Nutrition Pure Whey	130	26	1.5	1.5
Human Development Tech Solid Gains	694	60	100	6
Molecular Nutrition Sustained Protein	115	28.5	<0.5	<1
Sport Pharma Whey Protein Shake	120	24	2	3
Nature's Best Perfect Protein 92+	379	90.2	3.9	<1
Met-Rx Protein Plus	210	46	3	1.5
Cytodine Methoxy Pro	140	23	4	<1
Muscle Tech MASS Tech	830	45	150	6
Pro Lab 100% Pure Whey	130	22	6	2
Next Nutrition Designer Protein	90	17.5	3	1
Next Nutrition Big Whey	173	30	4.8	3.3
Vitol 100% Egg Protein	102	24	0	0
Note: All values listed based on serving size.				

Figure 3-4. Comparisons of various protein supplements

protein per serving (from various sources as well). For example, most pure protein powders contain approximately 100 to 250 kilocalories, 17 to 60 grams of protein, less than 6 grams of fat, and less than 6 grams of carbohydrates (not counting the macronutrients available in milk if the athlete uses milk as the liquid mix) (Figure 3.4).

Many multipurpose supplements (e.g., weight gainers, meal replacements) contain a larger amount of macronutrients (more than 600 kilocalories, more than 60 grams of protein, more than 50 grams of carbohydrates, and 6 to 20 grams of fat). Therefore, an athlete can easily obtain the recommended intake of protein via supplementation. Endurance training also increases protein requirements on a daily basis. High-intensity, long-duration aerobic training poses a great metabolic stress to the human body, resulting in substantial protein breakdown. Replenishing bodily protein stores is essential to recovery and performance. It is recommended that endurance athletes consume 1.4 grams per kilogram of body mass to offset the catabolic stress. Athletes deficient in protein intake may benefit the most from supplementation.

The timing of protein supplementation is important with respect to optimal recovery between workouts or competitions. Research has shown that consuming the supplement right after a workout or practice leads to an earlier increase in protein synthesis. In fact, postworkout supplementation is more effective following resistance exercise than a protein supplement taken hours later. Therefore, consuming a large amount of protein following training/competition (and maintaining adequate intake throughout the recovery period) is the most effective way to enhance recovery.

One concern with high levels of protein intake (and supplementation) is potential liver and kidney problems. For example, anecdotal reports suggest some athletes (especially bodybuilders and other athletes striving to maximize hypertrophy) consume protein well in excess of this recommended range. However, it is important to note that another factor affecting protein intake is the use of anabolic drugs (e.g., synthetic steroids, testosterone, and growth hormone), which increase the protein requirement. It is unclear, though, by how much, as science has not addressed this issue adequately. Therefore, drug-free athletes should not mimic the dietary strategies of an athlete who uses anabolic drugs because he will then run the risk of consuming too much protein. Protein supplementation within the recommended range appears safe and effective. Any intake beyond this level could increase the risk of problems, such as compromised kidney function and bone mineral loss.

Amino-Acid Supplementation

Amino-acid supplementation can increase protein synthesis following exercise, especially when carbohydrates are consumed simultaneously. The magnitude of the effect depends on:

- The dose of amino acids consumed
- The composition of the supplement (i.e., number and ratio of essential amino acids to nonessential)
- The timing of the supplement

The supplement dose and composition is important for increasing the availability of amino acids. Consuming an amino-acid supplement during the postworkout period speeds up the recovery process, which is of great importance to an athlete who has multiple competitions over the course of a week or on successive days. Low and high doses of essential and mixed amino acids (6 to 40 grams) increase protein synthesis substantially. Essential amino acids (especially BCAA) play a substantial role, as small doses lead to large elevations in protein synthesis. BCAA (especially leucine) directly increase protein synthesis. One reason for this increase is the anabolic hormone insulin, which increases proportionally to elevations in blood glucose and amino acids. Lastly, the timing of supplementation is important. Amino-acid uptake into muscle is greatest when blood flow increases. That is, taking a supplement in close proximity to the workout or practice session is very important to maximize amino-acid uptake. In fact, supplementing before the workout (and taking advantage of greater blood flow during the workout) increases amino-acid delivery to a greater extent than supplementing following the workout.

Amino Acids and Strength and Power Performance

Although amino-acid supplementation can enhance net protein balance following exercise, research does not support the contention that strength and power may be enhanced over time during training. Two studies (Antonio et al., 2000; Williams et al., 2001) have shown no further increase in muscle strength following six and 10 weeks of training. In a study we conducted, we did not see any further enhancement of strength or power with amino-acid supplementation following six weeks of training (four weeks of overreaching and a two-week taper phase) compared to a placebo. These results may be typical when the athletes are obtaining a sufficient amount of protein in their diets.

Individual Effects of Amino Acids

Besides being collectively included in protein or general amino-acid supplements, individual amino acids have been purported to have possible ergogenic effects on performance. The nature of these effects has been largely exaggerated in popular bodybuilding magazines. Although some investigations have demonstrated some potential positive effects, these results have been taken out of context and exaggerated

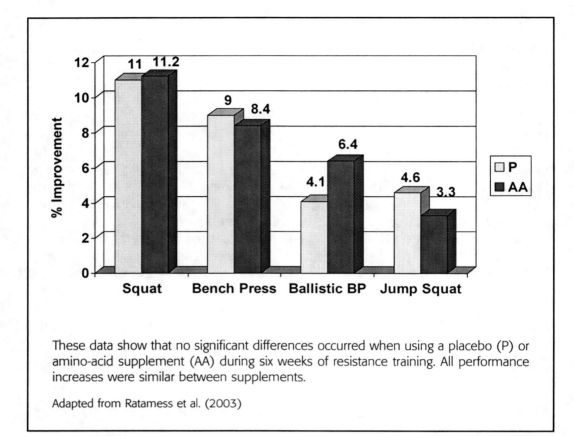

These data show that no significant differences occurred when using a placebo (P) or amino-acid supplement (AA) during six weeks of resistance training. All performance increases were similar between supplements.

Adapted from Ratamess et al. (2003)

Figure 3-5. Comparison of performance changes during six weeks of resistance training with amino-acid supplementation

with regards to the application of these findings to the athletic population. Some of the popular amino-acid supplements and purported claims include:

- Arginine—increased release of insulin and growth hormone, improved immunity, increased nitric oxide
- Lysine—increased growth-hormone release
- Aspartate—increased energy and endurance, reduced fatigue
- BCAA—reduced central fatigue (i.e., fatigue originating from the central nervous system), improved recovery, reduced protein breakdown, increased energy
- Glutamine—improved immunity and performance, increased muscle hypertrophy, enhanced recovery
- Ornithine—increased growth-hormone release
- Glycine—increased creatine phosphate synthesis, enhanced anaerobic performance

- Tryptophan—increased growth-hormone release, reduced pain, reduced central fatigue
- Tyrosine—increased adrenaline, strength, and energy
- Taurine—delayed fatigue, faster recovery, and antioxidant properties

Little scientific evidence is available to support supplementation with any of the individual amino acids other than BCAA, arginine, and glutamine. For example, some of the dosages that resulted in only slight elevations in growth hormone were far higher than those available in supplement form. Therefore, the athlete should supplement with protein and/or amino-acid supplements only when protein intake from dietary sources is inadequate.

Overreaching and Recovery

Overreaching occurs when the volume or intensity of training is increased greatly. The rationale is to "overwork" the body and then taper to produce a subsequent rebound in performance. Chronic overreaching can lead to overtraining, which is a syndrome characterized by performance reductions, among many other adverse effects. Therefore, a supplement that can reduce the negative impact of overwork (via better recovery) and maintain performance during these higher-volume phases (e.g., the in-season training period of athletes) could have a positive effect on performance. Because amino acids increase net protein balance, it has been suggested that amino-acid supplementation could improve recovery by reducing protein breakdown and potential muscle damage. Studies have shown that BCAA reduce protein breakdown and muscle damage in response to unaccustomed training. With this in mind, our laboratory group set out to investigate if amino-acid supplementation could provide some advantage during resistance-training overreaching.

In our study, we elicited overreaching by training all major muscle groups on consecutive days (to minimize recovery between workouts) and placed our subjects (resistance-trained men) into either an amino acid— or placebo-supplemented group. The amino-acid group consumed a mix of essential amino acids at 0.4 grams per kilogram of body mass per day. Each subject underwent four weeks of resistance training (after four weeks of low-volume, low-frequency base training), consisting of two two-week phases:

- Phase 1: three sets of eight- to 12-repetition maximum (RM) lifts for each of eight different exercises
- Phase 2: five sets of three- to five-RM lifts for each of five different exercises

In the placebo group, the athletes' 1-RM squat and bench press decreased after the first week (by 5.2 and 3.4 kilograms, respectively). Similar results occurred for upper-body power through the first two weeks. However, subjects in the amino-acid group maintained maximal strength and power despite the large physiological stress that occurred during the initial period of overreaching. Beyond the initial two weeks, 1-RM squat, bench press, and power increased similarly in both groups. We also included a subsequent two-week taper phase, which resulted in further strength gains in both groups, though amino-acid supplementation did not provide any further enhancement, as shown in Figure 3-5. The critical part of this study was the initial phase of training, which resulted in performance reductions and significant muscle damage in the placebo group only. Amino-acid supplementation reduced much of the damage, and the level of damage was related to the strength loss. We concluded that amino-acid supplementation was effective for maintaining performance during this period of unaccustomed, high-level training by enhancing the ability to recover between workouts.

Coaching Points

- Strength and power athletes should consume approximately 1.7 to 2.2 grams of protein per kilogram of body mass per day.

- Endurance athletes should consume 1.4 grams of protein per kilogram of body mass per day.

- Consuming a protein supplement immediately following a workout or competition is critical to optimizing recovery.

- Amino-acid supplementation does offset some of the negative effects of overreaching during high-volume strength training. However, it does not affect strength or power during normal training.

4

Lipids

ipids (from the Greek word *lipos*, which means fat) are fatty substances that do not dissolve in water. Lipids come in the form of oils (liquid at room temperature), fats (solid at room temperature), and other compounds. Lipids perform several functions critical to health and performance. *Glycerides*, the most common form of lipid, consist of a molecule of glycerol, which is bound to either one (*monoglyceride*), two (*diglyceride*), or three (*triglyceride*) fatty acids. Triglycerides account for approximately 90 percent of the lipids consumed by humans. Fatty acids may be saturated or unsaturated, with saturation referring to the number of hydrogen atoms bound to carbons in the fatty-acid chain. Therefore, *saturated fatty acids* contain no double bonds and hold the maximum number of hydrogen atoms. They tend to be solid at room temperature and are found in higher concentrations in animal products.

A *trans fatty acid* (which has a slightly different configuration than a saturated fatty acid) is an artificial fat found in many foods. Trans fatty acids may increase low-density lipoprotein (LDL) levels and increase the risk for heart disease. Unsaturated fats contain double bonds, which reduce the number of bound hydrogen atoms, and tend to be liquid at room temperature (e.g., various oils). *Monounsaturated fatty acids* contain one double bond, while *polyunsaturated fatty acids* contain two or more double bonds. The length of the fatty-acid chain also plays a key role in its function. Fatty acids with less than six carbons are *short-chain fatty acids*. Fatty acids with eight to 10 carbons are considered *medium-chain fatty acids*. The most abundant fatty acids are *long-chain fatty acids*, which contain more than 12 carbons.

Transport of lipids is also important once they are taken in through the diet. Short- and medium-chain fatty acids may be absorbed directly into the blood, but long-chain fatty acids (in addition to cholesterol and other phospholipids) need to be grouped together in the liver for transportation (e.g., the formation of a *lipoprotein*, which is a complex consisting of cholesterol, lipids, and protein). Different types of lipoproteins

Energy—Lipids are the most potent and concentrated macronutrient energy source. One gram of fat equals 9 kilocalories and provides more than 12 times the energy of 1 gram of carbohydrate. In addition, adipose tissue provides a large store of energy (i.e., subcutaneous body fat).

Essential Fatty Acids—Lipids provide essential fatty acids (i.e., linoleic acid, linolenic acid, oleic acid) necessary for bodily growth and function.

Fat-Soluble Vitamin Transport—Fat is necessary for the absorption of the fat-soluble vitamins A, D, E, and K.

Structural Components—Lipids make up cell membranes, nerve coverings, some hormones (e.g., cholesterol is a precursor of testosterone), and other substances vital to normal function.

Thermal Insulation—Body fat is essential to maintain normal body temperature.

Protection of Vital Organs—Essential body fat acts like a "shock absorber," as it surrounds major organs and protects them from damage during movement. Essential fat is about 3 to 4 percent of body mass in men and approximately 12 percent in women.

Figure 4-1. Functions of lipids

Fatty acid	Sources
Saturated fats	Meat, poultry, butter, cheese, whole milk, cream, cookies, crackers, chips, baked foods
Trans fats	Stick margarine, shortening, bakery items, candy, snack foods, fried foods
Monounsaturated fats	Oils: olive, canola, and peanut; nuts

Polyunsaturated fats
   Omega-6
 	
   Omega-3
	Oils: corn, safflower, sesame, soy, and sunflower; nuts
	
	Fish (herring, tuna, salmon, mackerel), canola and flaxseed oils, walnuts

Figure 4-2. Sources of dietary fat

exist in the human body. Low-density lipoproteins contain a high proportion of cholesterol and tend to clog the arteries with more regularity. High-density lipoproteins (HDL) contain more protein (and less cholesterol) and protect against cardiovascular disease by clearing the arteries. Cholesterol is a steroid precursor (i.e., a molecule needed to synthesize proteins) that also plays other significant roles in the human body. However, excessive cholesterol in the diet is a risk factor for cardiovascular disease.

Dietary Fat Intake

Adequate dietary fat intake is essential for an athlete, despite fat being demonized as something to be avoided at all costs. The prevailing thought among athletes has been to minimize fat intake as much as possible. However, reducing fat intake to below 15 percent of daily caloric intake may have negative consequences on endurance performance and reduce fat usage during exercise. Recommendations for athletes are similar to the recommendations for general health and fitness:

- Dietary fats should comprise 20 to 25 percent of total caloric intake.
- Less than 10 percent of fat kilocalories should come from saturated fats.
- Approximately 10 percent of fat calories should come from monounsaturated fats.
- Approximately 10 percent of fat calories should come from polyunsaturated fats, including at least 3 to 6 grams of essential fatty acids.
- Trans fatty acid consumption should be kept to a minimum.

Fat and Exercise

Fat is broken down from its storage sites and fatty acids are used for aerobic energy production. Triglycerides are stored in the liver, muscles, and adipose tissue. Muscle triglyceride stores are useful for immediate energy needs. Fatty acids from the liver or adipose tissue are broken down, enter circulation, and used for energy within the muscles during exercise. Fat is the predominant energy source in the human body during rest and low-to-moderate intensity exercise (i.e., up to 70 to 80 percent of $\dot{V}O_2$ max) of sufficient duration. The amount of fat utilized depends on the intensity and duration of the exercise session, as well as the diet and training status of the individual and the muscle-mass involvement. For example, higher rates of fat use are seen during running than during cycling.

For fat to be utilized efficiently during exercise, oxygen needs to be present in adequate quantities. Up to a certain point, when oxygen supply does not meet demand (i.e., anaerobic exercise), carbohydrates are the predominant energy source. This point varies from athlete to athlete, as an aerobically fit athlete can burn fat much more efficiently than an athlete with a lower level of aerobic fitness. In fact, maximal rates of fat oxidation occur at approximately 59 to 64 percent of $\dot{V}O_2$ max in trained individuals and at approximately 47 to 52 percent in lesser-trained individuals. Aerobic training leads to adaptations of skeletal and cardiac muscle (e.g., increase in $\dot{V}O_2$ max), as well as positive changes within the vessels and blood, which make it easier and more efficient to utilize oxygen and subsequently burn fat. Thus, the use of fat during aerobic exercise spares muscle glycogen and could enhance endurance performance. This information has served as the basis for investigating the use of fat supplementation for endurance performance.

Types of Fat Supplements

Based on the relevance of fat in human physiology, supplements have been developed with the notion of improving health and performance. Because of the role of fat in aerobic energy metabolism (and endurance performance), some experts have suggested that high-fat diets prior to an endurance workout/competition could enhance performance. Additional fat consumption (typically of long-chain fatty acids) is one method of supplementation. However, the size of long-chain fatty acids increases the time necessary for digestion, use, and absorption, in addition to creating a greater potential for storage if they are not oxidized. Medium-chain triglycerides have been used for supplementation to alleviate this problem. In addition, essential fatty acids have potential health-improving functions, which have led to the development of several supplements aimed at reducing body fat, reducing pain, improving oxygen delivery, and reducing the risk for cardiovascular disease.

High-Fat Diets

High-fat diets (more than 30 percent of daily caloric value) have been used by endurance athletes in an attempt to increase endurance during long-duration, low-to-moderate intensity aerobic exercise. The use of a high-fat diet as an ergogenic aid has been extensively questioned. The rationale for increasing fat consumption is based on attempts to spare muscle glycogen, increase fat usage (fat is a very concentrated energy source), and improve endurance performance. In fact, a high-fat diet (e.g., 85 percent of caloric intake) can reduce glycogen use and increase fat use to a much greater degree during exercise, but it also reduces muscle glycogen and increases muscle triglyceride levels prior to exercise. It is clear from the literature that substrate availability and use is dramatically altered with high-fat diets. However, the question of how these effects impact endurance performance has been more difficult to address, as some studies have shown enhanced endurance performance, while many others have shown no differences or even reductions in performance in response to high-fat diets (e.g., 38 to 85 percent of calories from fat) lasting seven to 49 days. In fact, studies that have examined short-term fat loading before exercise (46 to 94 percent of daily caloric value) have shown performance reductions during exercise of 68 to 75 percent of $\dot{V}O_2$ max as compared to high-carbohydrate diets.

Another concern with a high-fat diet is the potential for unwanted weight gain, increases in percent body fat, or elevations in blood lipids. Studies have shown that consuming 50 percent of calories from fat does not result in any further body-fat gain compared to a diet of 15 percent fat, and does not negatively affect blood lipid profile. Based on current research, it does not appear that high-fat diets have any more of an ergogenic effect on low-to-moderate intensity endurance performance than high-carbohydrate diets. From a coaching standpoint, it appears that consuming a diet high in carbohydrates (55 to 65 percent of caloric intake) as well as consuming fat in the desired range (e.g., 25 to 30 percent of caloric intake) is the best solution for the endurance athlete.

High-fat diets have no positive effect on high-intensity endurance exercise or anaerobic exercise in general. In fact, high-fat diets (42 to 67 percent of total caloric intake) have not been shown to affect endurance performance over 80 percent of $\dot{V}O_2$ max or enhance force production or power output. In contrast, a high-fat diet has been shown to reduce power output partially due to weight loss over time. High-fat diets, therefore, have no performance-enhancing potential for strength and power athletes.

Conjugated Linoleic Acid

Conjugated linoleic acid (CLA) refers to a group of positional and geometric isomers of an omega-6 fatty acid (linoleic acid) that have conjugated double bonds. CLA consists of different isomers, with the most common isomers in supplement form being the *cis*-9, *trans*-11 (c9;t11) and *trans*-10, *cis*-12 (t10;c12) isomers that constitute approximately 85 to 90 percent of the isomers used in supplements (*cis* and *trans* refer to the position of the double bond on the carbon chain). Most isomers are found in food, with higher concentrations found in ruminant meats (e.g., beef, lamb) and dairy products.

CLA supplements have been marketed to athletes with claims of reducing body fat, increasing lean-tissue mass, minimizing catabolism, and increasing strength and power. The basis of CLA claims derive from animal research in which CLA has been shown to decrease body weight, reduce body fat (via increase in fat oxidation, inhibition of fat storage, and reduction in fat-cell size), and increase energy expenditure. However, studies in humans have not consistently shown reductions in body fat. Studies in humans have typically supplemented the subjects with 1.7 to nearly 7 grams per day and conflicting reports of body-weight reduction and no changes have been shown. A recent study in resistance-trained men examined the effects of 6 grams of CLA per day for 28 days and found that CLA supplementation had no effect on body composition or muscle strength. Further research is needed to study CLA supplementation before conclusive evidence can be presented in support of CLA supplementation in athletes.

Medium-Chain Triglycerides

Medium-chain triglycerides (MCT), which have a length of six to 10 carbons, have been used to treat various ailments. In comparison to long-chain triglycerides, MCT are smaller in size, have a quicker transit time through the stomach, are more rapidly absorbed in circulation, and are not directly taken up into adipose tissue, as long-chain triglycerides are. Because of this, MCT have been regarded as supplements that could potentially reduce body fat and enhance endurance performance. However, many studies do not support these contentions. Supplementation with 25 to 50 grams of MCT consumed one hour before exercise has shown no effects on increasing blood fatty acids and sparing glycogen, and did not enhance exercise performance (dosing regimens higher than this have been shown to cause stomach distress and diarrhea). When carbohydrates are taken along with MCT, the addition of MCT does not have any effect over carbohydrates taken alone. Similar results have been obtained when MCT are taken during exercise. Thus, the results of these studies show that MCT do not enhance endurance performance in athletes and fail to provide support for MCT supplementation before and during exercise. However, some evidence does show that MCT may increase energy expenditure and reduce hunger. Therefore, MCT may have some role in weight loss, but further research is needed before any recommendations can be made.

Fish Oil Supplements

Fish oils and fish-oil supplements contain a substantial amount of the omega-3 fatty acids, eicosapentaenoic acid (EPA) and docosahexaenoic acid (DHA). Supplementation with omega-3 fatty acids has gained notoriety due to the positive health benefits associated with these fatty acids (e.g., reduced risk of cardiovascular disease, reduced LDL). Although omega-3 fatty acids have several health benefits, they do not appear to have any ergogenic effect on athletic performance. Studies have shown that omega-3 fatty acids (3 to 6 grams per day) do not enhance $\dot{V}O_2$ max or running performance in athletes or nonathletes. However, fish-oil supplementation has been shown to reduce exercise-induced bronchoconstriction in elite athletes, possibly due to an anti-inflammatory effect. Supplementation with omega-3 fatty acids does not enhance athletic performance. However, potential health benefits associated with omega-3 fatty acids make it attractive for supplementation.

Coaching Points

- Dietary fats should comprise 20 to 25 percent of total caloric intake, with less than 10 percent coming from saturated fats.
- No conclusive evidence exists to support CLA supplementation in athletes.
- MCT may play a role in weight loss, but they do not appear to enhance athletic performance.
- Fish-oil supplements appear to enhance health, but they provide limited ergogenic potential for athletes.

5

Vitamins, Minerals, and Antioxidants

Micronutrients (i.e., vitamins and minerals) are needed in small amounts in the human body (micrograms to milligrams per day). *Vitamins* are organic compounds essential for numerous bodily reactions to take place. They act as cofactors in many metabolic reactions and most need to be consumed in the diet for an individual to reach the RDA value. Thirteen vitamins are classified based on their solubility as either water- or fat-soluble. *Water-soluble* vitamins, which include the B vitamins and vitamin C, play major roles in energy metabolism and immune function. *Fat-soluble* vitamins, which include vitamins A, D, E, and K, are potent antioxidants and assist in recovery between workouts and practices. *Minerals* are inorganic compounds found in nature that are also essential to normal human functioning. Seven minerals are macrominerals (sodium, chloride, potassium, calcium, magnesium, phosphorus, and sulfur), because they are required in larger quantities. Others are microminerals required in small (trace) amounts.

The amount of vitamins and minerals consumed in the diet is critical to an athlete. Although vitamins and minerals are plentiful in food, vitamin/mineral content can be lost because of the way foods are processed, stored, and cooked. For example, cutting, cooking, freezing, heating, drying, and canning foods can reduce their nutritional value. Not only are some athletes' diets deficient in vitamin- and mineral-rich foods such as fruits and vegetables, but exercise and competition also increase the amount of vitamins and minerals needed on a daily basis. Studies in athletes show greater micronutrient turnover with high levels of physical activity, which results in additional loss of nutrients. Considering most young athletes' poor food selection and limited time for proper food preparation, vitamin/mineral supplementation appears very appealing. Vitamin and mineral supplements are commonly consumed by athletes. Some survey studies have shown that more than 50 percent (up to 85 percent) of athletes consume vitamin and mineral supplements, which are sold in the following ways:

- As a multivitamin/mineral supplement consisting of most, if not all, essential vitamin and minerals
- As a combo supplement consisting of a few synergistic micronutrients (e.g., B-complex)
- Added to other supplements (e.g., weight gainers, protein powders, all-purpose supplements)
- As individual vitamins or minerals (e.g., calcium, vitamin C)

The Rationale For Supplementing— Correcting the Dreaded Deficiency

The rationale for micronutrient supplementation is to correct possible deficiencies, which may lead to performance reductions and other serious health consequences. Vitamin/mineral supplements are not ergogenic in the sense that no additional performance enhancement will be observed with supplementation if sufficient amounts are consumed in the diet. Therefore, athletes who are nutrient-deficient (i.e., those who may be in weight-controlled sports, vegetarians, and those with poor diets) may benefit the most from supplementation. A deficiency may develop if an athlete only eats certain foods, has too low of a total caloric intake, or has a reduced ability to absorb vitamins/minerals due to other factors such as illness or drug or alcohol use. For example, many female athletes are deficient in calcium, zinc, and iron. Others have shown some deficiencies in thiamine, riboflavin, B6, and E. Correcting a deficiency takes some time. Therefore, frequent consumption of low doses of vitamins and minerals is a strategy used to prevent excessive excretion and correct a potential deficiency.

Working Together to Get the Job Done— Nutrient Synergy

Nutrient synergy is critical to micronutrient intake. Vitamins and minerals do not typically work independently. Instead, many interact with other vitamins and minerals, as well as with macronutrients. For example, large amounts of vitamin C may reduce copper utilization and increase iron absorption. Likewise, a deficiency in a vitamin or mineral could potentially limit the functioning of other micronutrients that are consumed in adequate amounts. Micronutrient intake should occur in balance with other micronutrients. This need for synergy is part of what makes multivitamin/mineral supplements so appealing, because the content typically reflects balance among micronutrients.

How Much Is Necessary?

Each vitamin and mineral is required in the body in different amounts. The latest method of rating dietary intake is the daily reference intake (DRI), which is an extension of the recommended daily allowance (RDA) and establishes the daily value that is necessary to maintain optimal health. The DRI also establishes a higher limit, which is important because consumption of more than this value may be common in populations that require more nutrients. In fact, athletes need more than the basic DRI values for most vitamins and minerals because of the stress of exercise and competition. How much more depends on several factors, including the intensity, volume, and frequency of exercise. Because of this variability, supplements become appealing if dietary intake is inadequate to meet the needs of training.

Vitamins

Thiamin (B1)

Thiamin plays a key role in carbohydrate and protein metabolism. From an athletic perspective, thiamin is essential to aerobic endurance. Good sources of thiamin include whole-grain cereal products, fortified bread, potatoes, legumes, pork, ham, liver, and nuts. The RDA for thiamin in adult men and women is 1.2 and 1.1 milligrams per day, respectively. Thiamin deficiency may result in loss of appetite, depression, weakness, and a nerve disorder called beriberi. Because thiamin is a vitamin needed for energy metabolism, its requirements increase in proportion to activity level. In fact, it is recommended that athletes consume 0.5 milligrams per 1000 kilocalories consumed per day. A few studies have shown that most athletes are not deficient in thiamin. However, the athletes most at risk tend to be those with limited caloric intake (e.g., those with weight classes, such as wrestlers and gymnasts). Thiamin supplementation is not recommended for athletes consuming a balanced diet. However, for athletes limiting caloric intake and consuming poor diets, a multivitamin supplement containing thiamin may be beneficial.

Riboflavin (B2)

Riboflavin plays a key role in energy (carbohydrate and fat) metabolism and helps maintain healthy skin and aerobic endurance. Good sources of riboflavin include dairy products, meat, eggs, green leafy vegetables, grains, and beans. The RDA for riboflavin is 1.3 and 1.1 milligrams per day for men and women, respectively, or 0.6 milligrams per 1000 kilocalories per day. A deficiency in riboflavin may result in dermatitis, oral sores, and eye damage. Most studies have shown that athletes are not typically deficient in riboflavin, though those with limited caloric intake may be at risk.

Riboflavin supplementation is not recommended for athletes consuming a balanced diet. However, for athletes limiting caloric intake or consuming poor diets, a multivitamin supplement containing approximately 100 percent of the RDA for riboflavin may be beneficial.

Niacin (B3)

Niacin (also called nicotinic acid) plays a key role in energy metabolism. In addition, niacin is thought to improve aerobic-endurance performance and increase blood flow to the skin, which helps with thermoregulation, especially during exercise in the heat. Good sources of niacin are meats, poultry, liver, fish, nuts, and grains. The RDA for niacin is 19 and 15 milligrams per day for men and women, respectively, and the upper-level intake per day is 35 milligrams. Niacin supplementation does not provide an ergogenic effect for athletes consuming a balanced diet. However, niacin consumed in higher amounts could lead to premature fatigue by reducing the amount of fatty acids available during exercise, thereby forcing the athlete to rely more on muscle glycogen. Overconsumption of niacin can also cause headaches, nausea, and itchiness. Most studies have shown that athletes are not typically deficient in niacin. Athletes most at risk are those with limited caloric intake. Niacin supplementation is not recommended for athletes consuming a balanced diet. However, athletes limiting their caloric intake or consuming poor diets may benefit from a multivitamin supplement containing approximately 100 percent of the RDA.

Pyridoxine (B6)

Vitamin B6 plays a key role in protein metabolism. It also plays a role in the formation of glucose, the breaking down of glycogen for energy, and the formation of hemoglobin and red blood cells. Vitamin B6 supplementation has been touted to increase muscle mass and strength and improve endurance. Good sources of B6 include meat, liver, poultry, fish, grains, bananas, green leafy vegetables, potatoes, and legumes. Although a B6 deficiency could hurt sports performance, most studies have shown no ergogenic effects when athletes consume a balanced diet. However, some studies have shown that 15 to 60 percent of athletes may have some deficiency in B6, which can result in anemia and nervous and muscular disorders. The RDA for B6 is 1.7 and 1.5 milligrams per day for men and women, respectively, and the upper level of daily intake is 100 milligrams. Therefore, supplementation is not recommended unless the athlete is in a weight-controlled sport or consumes a poor diet.

Folacin (B9)

Folacin (folate, folic acid) plays a key role in DNA and RNA metabolism and promotes hemoglobin and red blood cell formation. Theoretically, folacin has been touted to increase aerobic-endurance performance via replacement of red blood cells during exercise. Although a deficiency could hurt performance, studies have not shown any ergogenic effects of folacin supplementation on aerobic-endurance performance in athletes, despite elevations in the body's supply. A deficiency in folacin could lead to fatigue, anemia, and gastrointestinal problems. Good sources of folacin include meat, green leafy vegetables, liver, grains, potatoes, legumes, nuts, and fruit. The RDA for folacin is 400 micrograms per day for both men and women, but needs may increase during specific circumstances (e.g., pregnancy). Although some studies have shown athletes to be deficient in folacin, supplementation has not improved performance. Therefore, it is not recommended that athletes supplement folacin unless they are dietary-deficient.

Cyanocobalamin (B12)

Vitamin B12 plays a key role in DNA and RNA metabolism, promotes red blood cell production, and helps maintain nervous tissue. Vitamin B12 supplementation has been touted to increase muscle mass and strength and improve endurance. Although a B12 deficiency could hurt sports performance, research has not shown any ergogenic effects of B12 when athletes consume a balanced diet. A deficiency in vitamin B12 could lead to anemia, fatigue, and nerve damage. Good food sources of vitamin B12 include meat, fish, poultry, liver, eggs, and dairy products. The RDA for vitamin B12 is 2.4 micrograms per day for both men and women. Supplementation with vitamin B12 can be done through both oral and injectable means. Although some studies have shown athletes to be deficient in B12, supplementation with high doses (i.e., up to 1 gram per day) has not improved performance beyond that of normal intake. Therefore, it is not recommended that athletes supplement with vitamin B12 unless they are dietary-deficient.

A popular vitamin B12 supplement, especially among bodybuilders since the mid-1980s, is dibencozide. *Dibencozide* is the biologically active coenzyme of vitamin B12 (also called coenzyme B12) in the body and has been touted to build lean muscle mass (via increased protein synthesis) and reduce fatigue during exercise. Dibencozide was marketed as a legal "anabolic steroid replacer," suggesting that its use would produce gains in muscle size and strength similar to that of anabolic steroids. However, no studies have supported these claims. Therefore, it is not recommended that athletes supplement with dibencozide.

Pantothenic Acid (B5)

Pantothenic acid, another essential B vitamin, plays a key role in energy metabolism. Pantothenic-acid supplementation is thought to enhance aerobic-endurance performance. Although a deficiency could hurt sports performance, research has not shown any ergogenic effects of pantothenic acid when athletes consume a balanced diet. Although deficiencies are rare, a deficiency in pantothenic acid could lead to nausea, fatigue, and loss of appetite. Pantothenic acid is widely available in foods, including meat, liver, eggs, dairy products, grains, legumes, and vegetables. The RDA for pantothenic acid is 5 milligrams per day for both men and women. Supplementation with high doses (i.e., up to 2 grams per day) has not shown any ergogenic effect. Therefore, it is not recommended that athletes supplement with pantothenic acid.

Biotin (H)

Biotin plays a role in carbohydrate, fat, and protein metabolism, and studies show that biotin may regulate the expression of certain genes. The RDA for biotin is 30 micrograms per day for both men and women. Good food sources of biotin are meat, milk, eggs yolks, liver, grains, vegetables, and legumes. The body also has the ability to synthesize its own from bacteria in the gut. Biotin deficiencies may result in nausea, fatigue, skin problems, impaired immune function, and an accelerated aging process. Biotin is often found in lipotropic or "fat-burner" supplements due to its role in fat metabolism. An animal study showed that biotin supplementation increased lactate metabolism and resulted in higher levels of blood lipids (possibly via increased breakdown). However, no studies in humans have supported a fat-burning aspect to biotin supplementation. Therefore, it does not appear that biotin supplementation provides any benefits to athletes.

Choline

Choline is a "vitamin-like" compound that is sometimes included in "fat-burner" supplements because it plays a role in lipolysis, increases fat breakdown and transport for energy, and may promote preservation of the body's carnitine stores (carnitine is discussed in Chapter 10). By itself, choline supplementation does very little to reduce body fat. However, taken in conjunction with caffeine and carnitine, choline can reduce fat and improve aerobic-exercise performance in animals. Choline is a component of *lecithin*, which serves as a precursor for *acetylcholine*, a very important chemical messenger (called a neurotransmitter) in the body. Acetylcholine plays a critical role in transmissions from nerves to other nerves or skeletal muscles.

Theoretically, a higher content of acetylcholine could lead to enhanced neural function, strength, performance, and cognition. However, this theory does not appear to hold true. Although supplementation with lecithin can increase the synthesis of acetylcholine, no such ergogenic benefits have been found. A few studies examining marathon runners have shown that blood levels of choline are reduced by approximately 17 to 26 percent due to a greater metabolic need during exercise. Supplementation with lecithin (2.2 grams of choline) has been shown to actually increase blood choline concentrations following a marathon. However, the rise in blood concentrations has not had an ergogenic effect on performance during endurance exercise.

Primary dietary sources of choline include animal sources (e.g., meat, eggs), legumes, green vegetables, and nuts. A daily intake of 0.4 to 0.9 grams is sufficient to meet the body's needs. Some athletes supplement with choline at about 3 grams per day. However, choline supplementation is not recommended due to its lack of ergogenic effect on performance.

Inositol

Inositol is a B-complex-vitamin-like compound that has functions in metabolic regulation and growth. Inositol, like choline, is also included in many "fat-burner" or lipotropic supplements because it helps in the formation of lecithin, plays a part in the metabolism of fat and cholesterol, removes fats from the liver, assists choline in the formation of neurotransmitters, and may help control sugar cravings. Humans can make inositol in the body, and good dietary sources include fruits, lecithin, legumes, meats, milk, nuts, unrefined molasses, raisins, vegetables, and whole grains. No specific recommended intake is established for inositol. Most supplements include 250 to 800 milligrams. Signs of deficiency include high blood cholesterol, constipation, eczema, and hair loss. No ergogenic effects have been associated with inositol supplementation. Therefore, supplementation with inositol is not recommended.

Vitamin C (Ascorbic Acid)

Vitamin C, a major antioxidant, is one of the most popular vitamins supplemented by athletes. An antioxidant is a substance that limits the actions of *free radicals*, which are discussed later in this chapter. Free radicals cause damage to cells. Therefore, antioxidants are crucial to optimizing the function of the immune system and aid in recovery between exercise/competition bouts. In addition, vitamin C plays key roles in the formation of collagen (a very important structural protein for bones, tendons, and ligaments), wound healing, the development of connective tissue, iron absorption, and the formation of carnitine, red blood cells, and hormones such as steroids and catecholamines (adrenaline). Deficiency in vitamin C may result in muscle weakness, fatigue, infections, overtraining, increased risk of injury, anemia, bleeding gums, scurvy, and slow wound healing. Although a slight deficiency may not hurt performance in athletes, long-term inadequate intake can lead to these negative effects. Excellent food sources of vitamin C include citrus fruits, green leafy vegetables, potatoes, strawberries, broccoli, and green peppers. In addition, vitamin C is added to many products such as fruit juices, sports drinks, and other beverages.

As is the case with other vitamins, exercise and competition (in addition to extreme environmental temperatures, altitude, stress, and infection) increase the daily requirements of vitamin C for the athlete. Because of vitamin C's pertinent role as an antioxidant, maintaining adequate intake is essential to minimize the risk of upper respiratory tract infections (e.g., the common cold) and enhance recovery between workouts. Studies have shown that vitamin C supplementation significantly increases levels of vitamin C in blood and tissue, which could be important for offsetting the oxidative stress of free radicals during exercise and the subsequent recovery period. In fact, some studies have suggested that vitamin C supplementation can reduce the amount of muscle damage and thereby help maintain muscle strength and performance to a greater degree following unaccustomed exercise. It is important to note, however, that just as many studies have not shown those same effects. Acute supplementation with vitamin C does very little to help athletes. However, long-term supplementation (of at least 30 days) with vitamin C (especially in conjunction with other antioxidants such as vitamin E) appears to have a substantial effect in maintaining performance and enhancing recovery. These results show that to some extent, adequate vitamin C intake may enhance recovery in athletes, especially during times of high-volume, high-frequency activity.

Most studies show that vitamin C is not ergogenic, in that consuming more than the body needs will not result in any performance enhancement. In fact, vitamin C supplementation (beyond that of deficiency correction) does not enhance strength or endurance. However, supplementation with vitamin C may have greater importance to the athlete than what meets the eye. That is, by potentially enhancing recovery and immune function, adequate vitamin C intake may allow athletes to train harder and more frequently with lower incidences of upper respiratory infections (and subsequent reductions in missed or poor workouts), overtraining, and injuries. The recommended daily intake for men and women is 90 and 75 milligrams, respectively. However, athletes clearly require more, as reported intakes have ranged from 95 to 1,000 milligrams per day, with some athletes consuming well over 1,000 milligrams, especially during times of high stress. The upper limit for vitamin C intake is 2,000 milligrams per day, because long-term high intakes beyond this value could lead to kidney stones and gastrointestinal distress. Vitamin C supplementation may be necessary if an athlete's diet is deficient. Some experts recommend 500 to 1,000 milligrams per day for such athletes during periods of high-intensity and/or high-volume training or competition. Supplementation may be most beneficial when other antioxidants are supplemented in conjunction with vitamin C.

Vitamin A (Beta-Carotene, Retinol)

Vitamin A comes in many different forms. Preformed versions of vitamin A include *retinol*, *retinal*, *retinaldehyde*, and *retinoic acid*. In addition, many carotenoids are found in nature, at least 30 of which can be converted to vitamin A. These carotenoids are known as pro-vitamins. The most notable carotenoid is *beta-carotene*. For discussion purposes, all of these various forms will be referred to as vitamin A. Vitamin A plays key roles in vision, gene expression, maintenance of epithelial cells in the skin and mucous membranes, bone growth and development, and immune function. Like vitamin C, vitamin A is a critical antioxidant that may help in postworkout/competition recovery.

Deficiencies in vitamin A could lead to night blindness, dry skin, rough mucous membranes (and possible bleeding), poor immune function, and impaired growth and wound healing. It has been suggested that vitamin A, when consumed in adequate amounts, may reduce the risk of certain cancers. Excellent food sources of vitamin A include carrots, green leafy vegetables, spinach, tomatoes, oranges, apricots, broccoli, cantaloupe, sweet potatoes, liver, fish, dairy products, and eggs.

Vitamin A intake in athletes varies widely. Most studies have shown adequate intake in athlete, though some deficits have been shown in weight-controlled athletes (e.g., wrestlers, gymnasts), for whom intake was less than 70 percent of the RDA. In addition to low caloric intake, poor food selection (high in fat) and a lack of fruits and vegetables in the diet contribute to a deficiency. Because vitamin A is an antioxidant and is important for immunity and recovery, intake is related to activity level. Greater amounts are needed when the volume and intensity of training are high. Performance enhancement with vitamin A supplementation is not to be expected (unless it is taken in conjunction with other antioxidants). The recommended daily intake of vitamin A for men and women is 900 and 700 retinol equivalents, respectively (a retinol equivalent, or RE, is the standard unit of expression for vitamin A). Chronic high intake could lead to liver and kidney damage, hair loss, anorexia, fatigue, bone damage, headaches, joint pain, skin yellowing, and nausea. Because vitamin A deficiencies are not common (and a slight deficiency may not hurt athletic performance), supplementation is not recommended if the athlete consumes an adequate diet.

Vitamin D (Calciferol)

Vitamin D plays a key role in calcium and phosphorous absorption as well as in bone formation in the human body. Vitamin D is unique in that it can be produced in the body via ultraviolet light from the sun, which converts a skin compound called *7-dehydrocholesterol* into vitamin D. Slight modification to active vitamin D enables it to act in a way that is similar to a hormone when performing its primary role in calcium metabolism. A deficiency in vitamin D could lead to weak bones (i.e., rickets in children and osteomalacia in adults). The recommended daily intake for vitamin D is 5 micrograms for both men and women, and 10 micrograms per day for individuals under the age of 18. Some dietary sources of vitamin D include liver, fish, eggs, oils, margarine, and dairy products (fortified with vitamin D). Because of the amount of time an individual may be in the sun, the amount of vitamin D required from the diet varies. Although the skin adapts to chronic exposure to the sun by producing less of the vitamin D pro-vitamin (via tanning of the skin, use of lotions, aging), it is easier to attain adequate intake of this vitamin as compared to others. Vitamin D could be toxic at high levels, potentially leading to nausea, loss of appetite, joint pain, kidney damage, lethargy, and calcification of soft tissue. Because of its environmental abundance and the potential for toxicity, it is not recommended that athletes supplement with vitamin D.

Vitamin E

Vitamin E is the generic term for naturally occurring compounds called α-*tocopherols* and γ-*tocopherols* (the most common is *RRR*- or *d*-α-*tocopherol*). Vitamin E is a major antioxidant that prevents the destruction of red blood cells. Like vitamins C and A, vitamin E protects cells from free radical damage. Although rare, a deficiency in vitamin E could lead to anemia, red blood cell hemolysis, muscle and nerve damage, and inflammation. Good food sources of vitamin E include nuts, liver, eggs, vegetable and seed oils, and whole grains. The recommended intake for vitamin E is 15 milligrams (or 22 IU) per day for both men and women Note that 1 milligram equals approximately 1.5 international units (IU) of *d*-α-*tocopherol*. Intake should not surpass 1,000 milligrams per day, because long-term high intake could lead to headaches, fatigue, gastrointestinal distress, and greater risk of bleeding for those with clotting disorders.

Because of vitamin E's primary role as an antioxidant, athletes are particularly interested in the use of vitamin E supplements in enhancing recovery and limiting muscle damage between exercise bouts. The results of many studies have suggested that athletes may consume less than the recommended daily intake of vitamin E. For example, one study has shown that approximately 53 percent of college athletes consume less than 77 percent of the RDA. Therefore, vitamin E supplementation is quite common. However, the results of supplementation studies have been inconsistent. While both aerobic and anaerobic exercise have been shown to increase free radical activity and oxidative stress (via elevations in key blood markers), vitamin E supplementation has not been effective in reducing the total impact of the oxidative stress. In fact, only a few studies have shown reduced oxidative stress with vitamin E supplementation of up to 1,000 milligrams per day. In relation to performance, most studies have shown no ergogenic effects of vitamin E supplementation on muscle strength, endurance, and $\dot{V}O_2$ max. The exception is exercise studies conducted at altitude, which have shown vitamin E supplementation to be effective for enhancing exercise performance and $\dot{V}O_2$ max. Although the methods used in these studies are different and can be questioned, many experts believe that the results suggest that vitamin E works best in conjunction with other antioxidants rather than alone. Therefore, vitamin E supplementation may be useful for athletes who are deficient in their dietary intake. However, it appears vitamin E should be supplemented as part of a complete antioxidant supplement rather than by itself.

Vitamin K

Vitamin K plays a major role in blood clotting, glycogen and bone formation, and the synthesis of other proteins found in the blood, bone, and kidneys. Therefore, a deficiency could result in bleeding. Good food sources of vitamin K are liver, eggs, green leafy vegetables, tea, cheese, and butter. Vitamin K is also formed within the large intestine by beneficial bacteria. The recommended daily intake of vitamin K for men and women is 120 and 90 micrograms, respectively.

Very little is known about vitamin K in athletes. It has been shown that female endurance athletes who supplemented with vitamin K had a higher magnitude of bone formation than those who did not supplement. However, many of the women were deficient to begin with, so it appears supplementation corrected a deficiency. A follow-up study showed that vitamin K supplementation was not sufficient to offset reductions in bone mass observed in female endurance athletes over two years. Therefore, further work needs to be done to examine vitamin K supplementation in female athletes before any recommendations can be made. Because a deficiency in vitamin K is rare, it is not recommended that athletes supplement with vitamin K.

Minerals

Calcium

Calcium is a macromineral that performs a multitude of functions in the human body. Calcium promotes bone and teeth formation, mediates muscle contraction, is involved in nerve transmission, and regulates some enzyme activity. Good food sources of calcium include dairy products, egg yolks, beans, peas, dark green vegetables, and cauliflower. In addition, some beverages such as orange juice are fortified with calcium. The recommended dairy intake is 1,000 to 1,200 milligrams per day for both men and women, with an upper limit of 2,500 milligrams. Long-term excessive intake could lead to kidney stones, constipation, cardiac arrhythmias, and interference with the absorption of other minerals. A deficiency in calcium could lead to fatigue, muscle weakness, softened bones, and, in more serious situations, osteoporosis.

When athletes consume a balanced diet and meet their daily needs for calcium, any additional calcium intake does not have an ergogenic effect, but it may have a positive effect on maintaining good health. For example, one year of calcium supplementation at 1,000 milligrams per day has been shown to maintain and enhance bone mineral density in female distance runners during training. Athletes at risk may include those who have low dairy consumption, those consuming low-calorie diets, and perhaps aging athletes. Therefore, in most cases, calcium supplementation does not appear necessary from an ergogenic standpoint. However, from a health perspective, some groups of athletes (e.g., women, older athletes) may benefit from calcium supplementation of 500 to 1,000 milligrams per day.

Magnesium

Magnesium is a macromineral that plays key roles as a cofactor in more than 400 enzymatic reactions, including fat and carbohydrate metabolism and protein synthesis. Magnesium also impacts membrane stability and improves immune, neuromuscular, cardiovascular, and hormonal function. Good food sources of magnesium include green leafy vegetables, fruits, whole-grain products, milk, seafood, nuts, and yogurt. A deficiency in magnesium could result in muscle weakness, fatigue, cramps, muscle spasms, and poor performance, whereas chronic high intake could result in diarrhea, nausea, and vomiting. The recommended daily intake for men and women is 420 and 320 milligrams, respectively. Magnesium status in athletes has been shown to be variable. Overall, male athletes tend to consume enough in the diet (with the exception of those involved in weight-controlled sports), but female athletes tend to consume less than the recommended amount.

Diuretics and laxatives deplete magnesium in the body, so use of these substances is not recommended (athletes in weight-control sports tend to use them to make weight). Exercise can deplete magnesium levels as well, which prompts the use as of supplemental magnesium. In fact, supplementing with magnesium (250 to 500 milligrams per day) has been shown to reduce muscle damage, increase muscle strength and power, and improve endurance in a few studies in untrained individuals with unknown magnesium status. However, other studies have shown no such effects, probably because the athletes in these studies were not deficient in magnesium. When all of these studies are examined together, the consensus appears to be that magnesium supplementation has minimal effect on performance if dietary intake is sufficient. Therefore, supplementation is not necessary. The key for athletes is to consume somewhat more than the recommended amount from dietary sources because exercise/competition does increase magnesium requirements. However, if the diet is deficient, consuming magnesium as part of a multivitamin/mineral supplement may be helpful (e.g., 350 milligrams, or 100 percent of the daily recommended intake).

Sodium

Sodium is a macromineral that is typically very abundant in the American diet. Sodium maintains blood volume and fluid balance, and plays important roles in muscle contraction and nerve transmission. Sodium, along with potassium, is a major electrolyte, which means that it plays important roles in fluid balance, especially during exercise of prolonged duration in hot, humid weather, when fluid replenishment becomes a major concern. Much attention is given to excessive intake of sodium, which is common in the American diet. Chronically high sodium intake could lead to high blood pressure, which in turn could lead to cardiovascular disease. Although rare, sodium deficiency could lead to dizziness, muscle cramps, nausea, loss of appetite, and seizures. Sodium is found in abundance in many foods, including meat, fish, bread, canned foods, sauces, many "junk" foods, and table salt. The recommended daily intake range for sodium is 500 to 2,400 milligrams. Because of the abundance of sodium in the typical diet, supplementation is not necessary.

Chloride

Chloride is macromineral that plays a role in fluid balance and nerve function. Along with sodium, chloride is found in table salt. Excessive intake of chloride could lead to high blood pressure. Food sources of chloride include table salt, canned foods, meat, and fish. The recommended daily intake is 750 milligrams for both men and women. Because chloride is easily obtainable in the diet, supplementation is not recommended.

Phosphorous

Phosphorous is a macromineral that impacts bone formation, cell-membrane structure, energy production, acid buffering, and cell growth and repair. Good food sources of phosphorous include meat, eggs, fish, milk, cheese, grains, nuts, and legumes. The recommended daily intake is 800 to 1,200 milligrams for both men and women. A deficiency could result in muscle weakness, cramps, and weak bones, while chronic high intake could lead to impaired absorption of other key minerals. Phosphorous, in the form of several grams per day of phosphate salts, has been used for supplementation purposes. The rationale is phosphorous' roles in energy metabolism and its buffering ability. Phosphates are part of large energy sources in the body—ATP and creatine phosphate—that provide energy once they are biochemically cleaved. In cells, phosphates can buffer acids during exercise, thereby rendering it harmless and delaying fatigue. In addition, phosphates play a role in the formation of 2,3-diphosphoglycerate (2,3-DPG), which is located within red blood cells and facilitates the release of oxygen to working tissues. In theory, this effect could increase maximal aerobic capacity in an athlete. Some studies have shown promise, but others have not. In fact, phosphate loading (up to 4 grams per day, usually administered as 1 gram per dose four times daily) has been shown to improve $\dot{V}O_2$ max, exercise time to exhaustion, and 2,3-DPG concentrations, and improve markers of cardiovascular function in endurance athletes in some studies, but has had no effect on aerobic performance or power in others. It is difficult to determine the amount of ergogenic potential phosphate loading provides to the endurance athlete. Because some studies have found positive benefits with phosphate loading, more studies are warranted. For endurance athletes seeking to phosphate load, it appears that the protocols used in some of these studies may be beneficial (i.e., 1 gram dose taken four times per day for three to four days prior to the endurance event).

Potassium

Potassium is a macromineral that plays key roles in nerve conduction, muscle contraction, the establishment of normal membrane potentials, fluid balance, and the maintenance of normal heart rate, acid-base balance, protein metabolism, and carbohydrate metabolism. Like sodium, potassium is a major electrolyte in the human body and is prone to loss during prolonged endurance exercise, especially in hot, humid conditions. Good food sources of potassium include meat, fish, milk, yogurt, fruits, vegetables, potatoes, bananas, and bread. The daily recommended intake is 2,000 milligrams per day for men and women. A deficiency in potassium could lead to muscle cramps, loss of appetite, and an irregular heart beat, while too much potassium could lead to cardiovascular problems. Potassium intake beyond what the body needs is not ergogenic. Therefore, supplementation is not recommended when the athlete consumes adequate amounts in his diet. However, during prolonged exercise resulting in significant fluid loss, consuming potassium in a fluid-replenishment beverage is advantageous.

Iron

Iron is the most abundant trace mineral in the human body. It plays a key role in oxygen transport. The body contains about 3 to 5 grams of iron, as it serves as a functional component of proteins, including hemoglobin (approximately 60 to 70 percent), myoglobin (10 percent), and cytochromes (approximately 2 percent), which are involved in energy production. People typically lose 1 to 2 milligrams of iron per day. However, this value may exceed 7 milligrams per day in endurance athletes during periods of hard training.

Good dietary sources of iron include liver, eggs, meat, seafood, oysters, bread, legumes, nuts, green leafy vegetables, and broccoli. A key issue with iron intake is the amount that is actually absorbed. Iron bioavailability from meat sources (heme iron, which eventually forms hemoglobin and myoglobin) is relatively high, whereas absorption is relatively low from grains and vegetables (i.e., nonheme iron). In addition, vitamin C can help increase the absorption of nonheme iron in the diet. A deficiency in iron could result in fatigue and poor performance. More severe iron deficiency could result in anemia, which negatively affects health and performance. In fact, a deficiency in iron could limit aerobic metabolism and place greater emphasis on the glycolytic system. This effect may result in earlier onset of acidosis and premature fatigue.

The recommended daily intake for men and women is 18 and 8 milligrams, respectively. Male athletes tend to consume the recommended daily amount. However, female athletes tend to consume less than the recommended intake. In fact, iron deficiency is common in women in general, and the stress from exercise and competition simply exacerbates the problem. In addition to a lack of meat and iron-dense foods consumed in the diet, menstrual losses, the stress of exercise, loss in sweat and urine, gastrointestinal bleeding, and reductions due to repetitive trauma from contact with the ground (i.e., sports anemia) are all factors that lead to iron loss, especially in female endurance athletes. In fact, it has been reported that 25 to 44 percent of female runners are deficient in iron, while only 4 to 13 percent of male runners are iron deficient. Therefore, iron supplementation is common in female athletes and endurance athletes in general, especially for those with low intake of meat products. The effects of iron supplementation in athletes have been studied. In most cases, iron supplementation in athletes with only a mild deficiency or none at all has shown no ergogenic effects. However, numerous benefits have been observed in athletes with iron-deficient anemia. Studies have shown significant elevations in iron content in the blood (i.e., ferritin), as well as ergogenic effects such as improvements in exercise time to exhaustion, increased $\dot{V}O_2$ max, and reduced blood-lactate concentrations.

Endurance athletes, especially females, with iron deficiency should increase iron intake in the diet or consider supplementation. Iron supplementation of approximately 50 to 100 milligrams per day in endurance athletes with slight deficiencies has been recommended, while higher doses (up to 300 milligrams per day) have been recommended for athletes with severe anemia. Blood tests are commonly used to determine iron content, and serum ferritin levels of less than 35 micrograms per liter may necessitate iron supplementation. Supplementation is not necessary for athletes who are not deficient in iron, as chronic high iron consumption can lead to hemochromatosis (i.e., excess iron storage in the liver), heart disease, and liver damage.

Sulfur

Sulfur is a macromineral that plays a role in acid-base balance and connective-tissue structure. Considering that most sulfur in the body is found in the amino acids methionine, cystine, and cysteine, sources of sulfur are those foods that also provide adequate protein. Therefore, adequate protein intake ensures adequate levels of sulfur in the body. The effects of excess sulfur or a sulfur deficiency mirror those of protein.

Cobalt

Cobalt is a trace mineral that is a necessary component of vitamin B12. Cobalt is found in meat, liver, and milk. A deficiency could lead to anemia, while excessive intake could lead to nausea and vomiting. Cobalt needs are met when the athlete's vitamin B12 intake is adequate.

Copper

Copper is a trace mineral that is a component of many enzymes that are involved in normal iron absorption, energy metabolism, connective-tissue formation, and immune and cardiovascular function. A copper deficiency could result in anemia, whereas excessive intake could result in gastrointestinal distress. Food sources of copper include meat, fish, poultry, liver, eggs, nuts, legumes, and bananas. The recommended daily intake is 0.9 milligrams for both men and women, which can be easily attained through a balanced diet.

Iodine

Iodine is a trace mineral, the principle function of which is to serve as a component of the thyroid hormones—triiodothyronine (T3) and thyroxine (T4). The human body contains about 15 to 20 milligrams of iodine, 70 to 80 percent of which is found in the thyroid gland. Thyroid hormones are important for metabolic regulation and growth. A deficiency in iodine could lead to reduced metabolic rate and goiter (i.e., an enlargement of the thyroid gland), while excess intake could lead to impaired thyroid function. Food sources of iodine include iodized (table) salt, seafood, and vegetables. The recommended daily intake is 150 micrograms for both men and women, which is easily attainable through the diet.

Fluoride

Fluoride is a trace mineral that promotes the formation of bone and teeth. A deficiency in fluoride could lead to dental problems and perhaps a weakening of the bones. Sources of fluoride include seafood, milk, eggs, tea, and drinking water. The recommended daily intake for men and women is 4 and 3 milligrams, respectively. As water intake is critical to an athlete's diet, fluoride deficiency is not a problem.

Manganese

Manganese is a trace mineral that serves as a component of enzymes involved in energy and bone metabolism. A deficiency in manganese could lead to growth problems, while excess could lead to general weakness. Food sources include grains, peas, beans, nuts, leafy vegetables, and bananas. The recommended daily intake for men and women is 2.3 and 1.8 milligrams, respectively.

Molybdenum

Molybdenum is a trace mineral that is a component of enzymes involved in carbohydrate and fat metabolism. Sources of molybdenum include liver, grains, beans, and peas. The recommended daily intake is 45 micrograms for both men and women. Deficiencies are rare and athletes should have very little concern about molybdenum when consuming a balanced diet.

Selenium

Selenium is a trace mineral that plays a very important role as a cofactor with the enzyme *glutathione peroxidase* and works in synergy with vitamin E. In both cases, selenium acts as an antioxidant that aids in enhancing immune function and recovery ability. A deficiency in selenium can lead to immune dysfunction, fatigue, impaired recovery, cardiac problems, and potentially cancer, while an excess can lead to gastric distress and fatigue. Good food sources of selenium include meat, liver, poultry, fish, seafood, dairy products, nuts, and grains. The recommended daily intake of selenium for men and women is 70 and 55 micrograms, respectively.

Because of its role as an antioxidant, selenium supplementation can be enticing, especially for athletes striving to enhance immune function, reduce muscle damage, and improve recovery between workout sessions or competitions. Some studies have examined selenium supplementation of 100 to 180 micrograms per day as part of an antioxidant cocktail and have shown glutathione peroxidase activity to be increased, which is suggestive of enhanced antioxidant functioning. However, no ergogenic effects on performance have been found. Therefore, selenium supplementation for athletes who obtain a balanced diet and proper kilocalorie intake is not necessary. However, because exercise increases the need for selenium and some athletes have poor diets and require strict weight control, selenium supplementation of less than 100 micrograms per day as part of an antioxidant supplement may be beneficial.

Chromium

Chromium is a trace mineral that is also a popular supplement targeted to athletes seeking to increase muscle mass. Chromium's primary role is to augment the action of the hormone insulin (as part of a complex known as the *glucose tolerance factor*), and it therefore plays a role in carbohydrate, protein, and fat metabolism. Insulin assists with the transport of glucose and amino acids into the cells and is a potent anabolic hormone that increases protein synthesis (and slows protein breakdown). In theory, by increasing insulin sensitivity, chromium supplementation could enhance lean body mass and reduce body fat. In addition, it has been shown to lower blood cholesterol. In fact, chromium has been used in diabetic populations to lower blood sugar levels. Food sources of chromium include whole grains, cheese, nuts, mushrooms, asparagus, and some meats. The recommended daily intake for men and women is 35 and 25 micrograms, respectively. Chromium deficiency could lead to glucose intolerance and impaired fat metabolism.

Potential ergogenic effects of chromium supplementation have been studied since the late 1980s. Supplementation with chromium occurs primarily in the form of chromium picolinate, as this form increases the amount of chromium absorbed and is considered to be most effective. Most chromium picolinate supplement studies used 60 to 1,000 micrograms per day for six to 38 weeks. A few early studies showed increases in lean body mass and loss of fat with 200 micrograms of chromium picolinate per day. However, the body-composition measurement methods used in those studies have since been challenged (and diet was not controlled for).

Approximately 10 to 15 percent of subsequent studies have shown greater increases in lean body mass with 200 to 400 micrograms per day, but the majority of studies have produced no additional improvement. In fact, subsequent studies have shown no effect on lean-tissue mass, fat mass, or muscle strength in weight-trained men, women softball players, Division I NCAA wrestlers, and American football players. In fact, statistical evaluation of the studies examining chromium supplementation has shown a slight effect, at best, on body composition in healthy adults and athletes. Therefore, the ergogenic evidence is not convincing enough to support the use of chromium picolinate supplementation. However, exercise and competition increase chromium requirements and some athletes may have some deficiency that could warrant supplementation. A safe and recommended supplementation intake is 50 to 200 micrograms per day for athletes thought to have a deficiency. Consuming more than 200 micrograms leads to substantial excretion of chromium. Many supplements have used a niacin-based chromium mixture, *chromium polynicotinate*. This form is considered to be as good as, or even better than, chromium picolinate because of a greater amount of chromium absorbed when it is bound to niacin, though little is known about this mixture and its affect on athletic performance.

Zinc

Zinc is a major trace mineral that is involved in a multitude of functions. Approximately 86 percent of the zinc in the body is found in skeletal muscle and bone. Zinc is an essential component of several hundred enzymes that catalyze numerous reactions in the human body. In addition, more than 200 zinc-dependent transcription factors (necessary for gene expression) have been identified. Therefore, zinc plays critical roles in protein synthesis, tissue repair, recovery, glucose metabolism, hormone metabolism (i.e., elevation of blood testosterone), bone development, and wound healing. In addition, zinc plays a substantial role in immune function and is a structural element of *superoxide dismutase (SOD)*, which is an antioxidant.

A deficiency in zinc could result in impaired growth, reduced work and power capacity, higher blood lactates during exercise, impaired immune function, and greater muscle damage. Chronic high intake of zinc could lead to anemia, gastrointestinal distress, and poor absorption of other minerals such as iron and copper. Good food sources of zinc include beef, shellfish, oysters, red meats, eggs, liver, whole grain cereals, nuts, and legumes. Meats, liver, and eggs are considered especially good sources because more zinc is absorbed after they are consumed. The recommended daily intake for zinc for men and women is 11 and 8 milligrams, respectively.

Dietary intake of zinc has been shown to be deficient in several groups of athletes. In fact, estimates show that as many as 90 percent of the athletes tested in studies had lower consumption of zinc than the recommended minimal intake. Athletes at risk tend to be endurance athletes, athletes who need to compete in weight classes, and athletes with high-carbohydrate, low-protein, and low-fat diets. In fact, food restriction and poor diet (i.e., low protein intake) are the major factors contributing to zinc deficiency.

Physical activity requires more zinc in the diet because zinc is excreted in sweat and redistributed between the red blood cells and the blood plasma. Zinc supplementation can benefit athletes who have a deficiency by restoring muscle strength and endurance. In fact, supplementation with zinc improves immune function; reduces free radical damage; improves muscle strength, endurance, and exercise tolerance; and reduces blood viscosity in individuals who most likely had a deficiency. Therefore, zinc supplementation is not necessary for athletes who consume a balanced diet with adequate protein intake (and consumption of animal products). However, athletes who may be deficient may benefit from supplementation (as part of a multivitamin/mineral supplement) of 11 to 15 milligrams per day. Supplementation should not exceed 50 milligrams per day, as this intake level can interfere with iron and copper absorption.

In supplement form, zinc has been combined with magnesium into a product known as ZMA. The combination is thought to enhance the anabolic hormonal responses to training. One study (Brilla and Conte, 2000) has examined the effects of this supplement on football players and found that the players taking ZMA (30 milligrams of zinc monomethionine aspartate, 450 milligrams of magnesium aspartate, and 10.5 milligrams of vitamin B6) had greater strength improvements and higher blood concentrations of testosterone and IGF-1 (two anabolic hormones that cause muscle growth). Note that the inclusion of vitamin B6 and the aspartate complexes was used to increase mineral absorption. While these results look promising, further research is needed before any recommendations can be made regarding supplementation with ZMA.

Boron

Boron is a mineral that has received some attention in the supplement industry, especially among bodybuilders. Boron has been shown to affect the metabolism of other macrominerals such as magnesium, phosphorous, and calcium, therefore suggesting a possible role in bone metabolism. However, its popularity is based on claims that it could increase testosterone concentrations. These suggestions were based on early reports that suggested that postmenopausal women had higher testosterone concentrations (as well as estradiol) following boron supplementation. However, a study (Green and Ferrando, 1994) in bodybuilders was conducted in which male bodybuilders were given 2.5 milligrams of boron or a placebo for seven weeks. The researchers found no differences in lean body mass, one-repetition maximum bench press or squat performance, or testosterone concentrations between the groups, despite increases in blood boron concentrations.

Another study supplementing healthy men with 10 milligrams of boron per day showed small, transient elevations in testosterone, but estradiol increased as well (i.e., resulting from aromatization of testosterone). Therefore, oral supplementation in athletes appears to have no ergogenic benefits, despite some transient elevations in testosterone found in one study. Based on current data, boron supplementation is not recommended for athletes. Food sources of boron include leafy vegetables, fruits, nuts, and legumes. Boron is also found in significant concentrations in some alcoholic beverages. Most individuals consume about 0.3 to 4 milligrams of boron per day. Although no RDA is provided for boron, obtaining 1 to 2 milligrams of boron per day is easily done through a balanced diet.

Vanadium

Vanadium is another trace mineral that has received attention in the supplement market (*vanadyl sulfate*). Although numerous functions for vanadium have been proposed, its chief role for supplementation purposes entails its insulin-like properties. Insulin is a hormone that is very important for enabling glucose and amino acids to enter the cells. Therefore, insulin is a potent anabolic hormone, and because of vanadium's similar role, supplement companies have touted vanadyl sulfate as an anabolic supplement and targeted it especially to bodybuilders. Although some studies have shown a potential insulin-like action of vanadium in animals and humans (especially obese, diabetic populations), the evidence in athletes does not demonstrate a clear rationale for use. One study (Fawcett et al., 1996) examined 12 weeks of vanadyl sulfate supplementation (0.5 milligrams per kilogram of body weight per day, or approximately 40 milligrams) and reported no ergogenic effects on body composition or most strength measurements. Because of the lack of data supporting its use, supplementation with vanadyl sulfate is not recommended.

Deficiencies in vanadium are rare and an athlete can certainly attain adequate amounts from a balanced diet. Food sources of vanadium include shellfish, mushrooms, black pepper, and parsley, and smaller amounts are found in fruits and vegetables. Although no recommended level has been established for vanadium, it appears that intake of up to 100 micrograms per day is common. Some bodybuilders consume in excess of 150 milligrams per day. However, this level of intake should be not be allowed among your athletes, as this amount of vanadium can be toxic and lead to liver damage and gastrointestinal problems.

Other Antioxidants

Antioxidants, which include the previously discussed vitamins A, E, and C, and the mineral selenium, play major roles in the human body. It is important to understand the function of antioxidants and describe some other key antioxidants needed for optimal health and performance.

Atoms tend to be in a "grounded" state in which every electron in the outer shell has a complimentary pair. A *free radical* has at least one unpaired electron and is highly reactive. When a free radical involves oxygen, it is known as a *reactive oxygen species*

(ROS) and will "steal" electrons from cell membranes, which have an abundance of polyunsaturated fatty acids. This process is known as *lipid peroxidation* (i.e., a free radical attack) and will propagate from molecule to molecule, causing more damage. The most common ROS are superoxide anion, hydroxyl radical, singlet oxygen, and hydrogen peroxide. In fact, up to 5 percent of the oxygen an individual consumes at rest during or exercise becomes damaging free radicals. Therefore, free-radical damage (via lipid peroxidation) occurs when free-radical production exceeds the body's ability to control its activity (a scenario known as *oxidative stress*).

Control is supplied by the antioxidant defense system. Exercise and the stress of competition increase free-radical production, which ultimately could lead to tissue damage, injury, and fatigue. Antioxidants protect tissues by donating an electron to the free radical, thereby rendering it harmless. Oxidative stress occurs in all athletes, but the magnitude may be worse in lesser-trained individuals. As an adaptation, the human body has the ability to lessen the magnitude of free-radical damage, either by reducing free-radical production or by upregulating antioxidant enzymes.

Dietary antioxidant intake is critical to upregulating the body's antioxidant defense system. The human body contains three major enzymes that are used to neutralize free radicals: *superoxide dismutase (SOD)*, *catalase*, and *glutathione peroxidase*. Consumption of antioxidants from dietary sources or through supplementation helps the body increase the ability to neutralize free radicals. Some supplements contain these compounds. However, it is questionable as to how well they are absorbed and just how much the body can utilize. Therefore, the best strategy for athletes is to consume dietary sources of antioxidants and, if necessary, a balanced antioxidant formula to optimally neutralize free-radical damage. The following antioxidants have been customarily found in supplements:

- *Glutathione* is an enzyme cofactor formed in the liver from the amino acids cysteine, glutamic acid, and glycine, which form the antioxidant enzyme glutathione peroxidase as well other enzymes. Glutathione is also thought to conserve other antioxidants such as vitamins A and E. Although glutathione is synthesized within the body, the stress of exercise/competition and amino-acid deficiencies in the diet can deplete glutathione. Although no recommended intake is provided for this substance, some supplements have included 12.5 to 250 milligrams (of L-glutathione) to be taken on a daily basis.

- *N-acetyl-cysteine (NAC)* increases glutathione concentrations in the blood. Although no recommended intake is provided for this substance, some supplements have included 50 to 200 milligrams of NAC.

- *Alpha lipoic acid (ALA)* has antioxidant functions and may increase glutathione levels, but it also acts as a cofactor in energy metabolism and may increase the effectiveness of other vitamin antioxidants. Although no recommended daily intake is provided for this compound, supplements usually contain 50 to 300 milligrams of ALA.

- *Lycopene* is a carotenoid found in fruits and vegetables that has potent antioxidant function. Although no recommended daily intake is provided for this compound, supplements usually contain 3 to 10 micrograms.

- *Coenzyme Q10 (ubiquinone)* is found in beef, chicken, pork chops, and salmon. Coenzyme Q10 is involved in energy production, but also acts as an antioxidant in defending the body from free radicals. Although no recommended daily intake is provided for this compound, supplements usually contain 10 to 130 milligrams.

- *Pycnogenol* is an antioxidant derived from pine bark extract. Although no recommended daily intake is provided for this compound, supplements usually contain approximately 50 milligrams.

- *Grape seed extract* is a potent antioxidant thought to protect connective tissue from free-radical damage. Although no recommended daily intake is provided for this compound, supplements usually contain 50 to 100 milligrams.

Coaching Points

- The rationale for vitamin and mineral supplementation is to correct possible deficiencies. If no deficiency exists, supplementation is not necessary, as consumption of additional amounts is not ergogenic.

- Vitamins and minerals work in synergy; therefore, balance in consumption is necessary.

- Training and competition increase vitamin/mineral requirements above the recommended daily intake.

- B-complex vitamins are critical for energy metabolism and are required in ranges from 1.1 to 1.7 milligrams per day (thiamin, riboflavin, pyridoxine), 5 milligrams per day (pantothenic acid), 15 to 19 milligrams per day (niacin), and in smaller amounts for cyanocobalomin (2.4 micrograms per day) and folacin (400 micrograms per day).

- Vitamin C is an important antioxidant required in a range of 75 to 90 milligrams per day. Supplementation with up to 2000 milligrams per day is common in athletes.

- Fat-soluble vitamins have important antioxidant functions and are required in ranges of 5 micrograms per day (vitamin D), 90 to 120 micrograms per day (vitamin K), 15 milligrams per day (vitamin E), and 700 to 900 retinol equivalents (RE) per day (vitamin A).

- Macrominerals perform a multitude of functions and are required in ranges of 8 to 18 milligrams per day (iron and zinc), 320 to 420 milligrams per day (magnesium), and 500 to 2000 milligrams per day (sodium, chloride, phosphorous, calcium, and potassium).

6

Creatine

Creatine is one of the most commonly used supplements among athletes. Since the early 1990s, creatine supplementation has been a hot topic in sports science after some initial research showed its ergogenic potential. Many studies have since been published and many athletes have supplemented with creatine. Some notable professional athletes have also endorsed creatine, which has contributed to its popularity. In contrast to some of the other supplements discussed in this book, creatine has been scientifically shown to be an effective ergogenic aid, although the long-term health effects remain unknown.

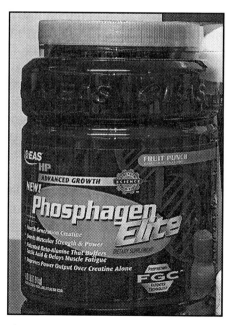

Figure 6-1. Creatine supplement

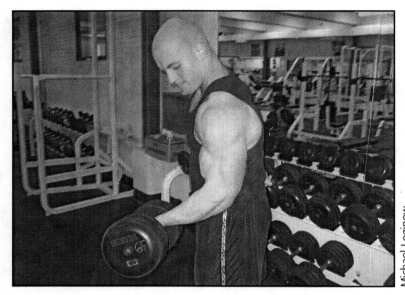

Figure 6-2. A strength athlete who would benefit from creatine supplementation

Creatine's Physiological Value

Creatine, a nitrogenous amine, was discovered by a French scientist named Michel Chevreul in 1832. However, the idea for supplementation did not develop until much later. The rationale for creatine supplementation stems from its role in anaerobic energy metabolism and its ability to act as an osmotic agent. The human body possesses three basic energy-producing systems, an aerobic energy system and two anaerobic systems. The body's basic energy unit is *adenosine triphosphate (ATP)*. The anaerobic energy systems provide energy liberation during high-intensity exercise. Although humans are capable of storing a small amount of ATP, this amount only provides enough energy for one to two seconds of activity. Therefore, the body constantly needs to resynthesize ATP for energy use, and creatine phosphate plays a vital role in the resynthesis of ATP. Creatine phosphate (CP) is a high-energy phosphate compound that is very important during high-intensity activities that require maximal effort for a short period of time. The CP system (also called the phosphagen system) can supply energy for activities for approximately 10 to 15 seconds before substrate depletion.

The CP reaction looks like this:

$$H^+ + CP + ADP \leftrightarrow ATP + Cr$$

This reaction is catalyzed by an enzyme called creatine kinase. The quick, high-energy burst needed for sprinting, lifting weights, or explosive jumping is provided to athletes predominantly via the ATP-CP system. Critical to this bioenergetic pathway is the ability to quickly resynthesize CP for further high-energy bouts of exercise, as high-intensity exercise may deplete CP by 70 percent during the first 30 seconds. Luckily, this reaction is reversible, so that creatine can be rephosphorylated to CP for energy. Within 20 seconds, 50 percent of CP is restored; within 40 seconds, 75 percent is restored; within 60 seconds, 87 percent is restored; and nearly all CP is restored within three minutes of recovery. The process of ATP formation also buffers ADP, which has been shown to be a factor in fatigue. Therefore, the rationale to supplement with creatine relates to the potential to increase muscle concentrations and have faster resynthesis during recovery, which improves high-intensity exercise performance. These effects enhance an athletes' quality of training and result in a greater volume of training in a particular time interval.

A second major factor is that creatine acts as an osmotic agent within skeletal muscle. When muscle creatine stores increase, this process attracts water to enter the cells via a process called *osmosis*. This initial water retention has potential benefits. For example, creatine supplementation has been shown to increase body weight. In fact, athletes beginning a creatine supplementation phase may gain weight after just a few days. Is this weight gain in the form of muscle mass? Initially, the answer is no. However, studies have shown that an increase in intracellular water concentrations leads to increased protein synthesis and muscular growth, which means that although the initial weight gain with creatine supplementation is predominantly due to water retention, this process ultimately leads to an increase in muscle mass. This benefit also provides another explanation regarding the ergogenic effects of creatine, but it could also pose a problem to some athletes who are in weight-controlled sports, as weight gain may not be an immediate desired effect. In addition, most studies show that creatine supplementation can enhance muscle glycogen stores as well, which can have a substantial impact on high-intensity muscular endurance, as muscle glycogen levels can become depleted over time during high-intensity exercise.

Creatine Requirements and Food Sources

Creatine is naturally found in foods, but it also is synthesized in the human body from the amino acids arginine, glycine, and methionine in a couple of different reactions. Creatine is metabolized to creatinine, which is excreted in urine at a rate of approximately 1.6 percent of total creatine stores in the body per day. Through endogenous synthesis (i.e., synthesis within the body) and diet, creatine needs are estimated to be approximately 2 grams per day for an average-sized (70 kilogram) man. Consumption of this amount is easily achievable through diet and supplementation. Creatine is found in high concentrations in meat and fish. For example, an athlete could get 2 to 3 grams of creatine simply by consuming 1 pound of beef, herring, tuna, or salmon. However, larger amounts are typically consumed via supplementation (5 to 20 grams). Although no specific recommendation has been made for daily creatine intake, athletes involved in anaerobic sports would benefit from consuming at least 2 to 3 grams per day to increase muscular concentrations of creatine.

Creatine Absorption and Storage

Creatine is absorbed through the small intestine and enters the bloodstream, where it circulates throughout the body. Although creatine is absorbed in other tissues (e.g., the brain and heart), approximately 95 percent of creatine is absorbed in skeletal muscle. The process of tissue creatine transport is rather interesting. A specific creatine-transporter protein located within the muscle's cell membrane helps creatine enter the muscle. When elevated levels of creatine are present in the blood, creatine (along with sodium and chloride) is actively transported into skeletal muscle, thereby increasing muscle creatine content. The extent of the increase depends on the fiber type and the initial level of creatine in the muscle. Interestingly, this transporter's expression (or activity) is greater during times of creatine deficiency, and is higher in slow-twitch muscle fibers, which store less creatine than fast-twitch fibers (which is the opposite of what might be expected). The regulation of this transport protein is important when considering supplementation. It is thought that an increase in creatine levels negatively impacts the transporter, thereby establishing a limit on how much creatine the muscles can store. In animals, this transporter is downregulated with creatine loading, though this effect may not be present in humans. In either scenario, this transporter's activity may pose a limit to how much creatine can be stored in muscles during supplementation. Most creatine (60 to 70 percent) entering the muscle is trapped by phosphorylation to creatine phosphate (by ATP), thereby exhibiting its role as a high-energy phosphate.

Muscle Creatine and the Influence of Supplementation

Creatine supplementation can substantially increase muscle levels of total creatine (creatine and CP). Overall, the total muscle creatine content is about 120 to 125 millimoles per kilogram of dry weight under normal circumstances. A study by Harris et al. (1992) examining creatine loading and subsequent maintenance doses showed that creatine supplementation could increase muscle creatine content to 155 millimoles per kilogram of dry weight. Several subsequent studies have shown significant increases in muscle creatine content following supplementation. In fact, the range of increases has been between 11 and 22 percent in most cases. The majority of muscle creatine elevation occurs within the first few days of supplementation, after which a plateau is achieved. Further supplementation with lower doses has been

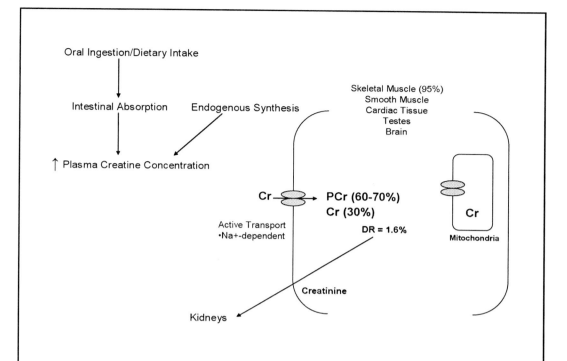

Oral Ingestion/Dietary Intake

Intestinal Absorption   Endogenous Synthesis

Skeletal Muscle (95%)
Smooth Muscle
Cardiac Tissue
Testes
Brain

↑ Plasma Creatine Concentration

Cr ⟶ PCr (60-70%)
Cr (30%)

Active Transport
•Na+-dependent

DR = 1.6%

Cr

Mitochondria

Creatinine

Kidneys

Once creatine is ingested, it is absorbed through the lumen of the small intestine, which subsequently leads to an increase in creatine levels in the blood. Creatine is taken up into muscle via membrane-bound transporters, which also require sodium and chloride to form a gradient to assist in creatine transport. Approximately 60 to 70 percent of creatine is phosphorylated to CP, which can be used to meet high energy needs. Creatine is degraded at a rate of 1.6 percent per day to creatinine in the kidneys, where it is excreted. In addition, creatine is thought to be "shuttled" to mitochondria, where it can be resynthesized to CP and used in the cytoplasm to meet high energy demands.

Figure 6-3. Creatine kinetics

shown to maintain this higher level of creatine content. It is important to note that most studies have incorporated a "loading" phase, which consists of 20 to 30 grams per day for five to seven days, followed by a maintenance dose ranging from 2 to 5 grams per day for several days. The largest increases have been shown in subjects with initially low levels of creatine. It appears that approximately 150 to 160 millimoles per kilogram of dry weight may be the ceiling limit for muscular creatine content. Once this ceiling limit is reached, higher doses will not increase creatine content any further. However, not everyone attains this level. Some individuals (i.e., nonresponders) attain little to no increase, while some people experience very large elevations.

Factors Influencing Creatine Uptake

In addition to the activity of creatine transport proteins, other factors may influence how much creatine can be stored in skeletal muscle. First, initial creatine content is a key. Individuals with lower levels of creatine have shown greater rates of uptake than those with higher levels. This response is particularly evident with vegetarians, who typically have lower levels of muscle creatine due to lack of animal sources in their diets. Another key factor is the muscle fiber type. Fast-twitch muscles (i.e., anaerobic fibers vitally important for strength and power activities) can store more creatine than slow-twitch endurance fibers, which is important because creatine is an ergogenic supplement when it comes to enhancing anaerobic performance. Therefore, having greater potential to store creatine in fast-twitch fibers is an advantage. Creatine supplementation, in combination with an exercise program, is more effective for increasing creatine uptake than supplementation alone. In addition, uptake is much greater when creatine is ingested along with carbohydrates than when creatine is consumed alone. Green and colleagues (1996) showed that consuming 5 grams of creatine plus 90 grams of glucose increased creatine content much more than consuming the creatine alone. In response to these findings, many creatine supplements on the market contain carbohydrates to maximize uptake. It is thought that exercise and creatine-plus-carbohydrates in combination may increase uptake to an even greater extent, possibly due to some insulin-mediated mechanism.

Another factor affecting creatine's ergogenic potential is its use in combination with caffeine. Conflicting reports have been published in this area. Creatine and creatine + caffeine (5 milligrams per kilogram of body mass per day) resulted in similar elevations in CP in one study (Vandenberghe et al., 1996). However, the rates of CP resynthesis were slightly impaired when caffeine was consumed with creatine, and additional performance enhancement brought about via creatine supplementation was negated when caffeine was consumed in conjunction. In addition, Hespel et al. (2002) showed that creatine supplementation reduces muscle relaxation time by 5 percent (which may positively affect some aspects of performance), though consumption of 5 milligrams per kilogram of body weight per day of caffeine eliminated this ergogenic effect of creatine. In contrast, Doherty and colleagues (2002) supplemented trained men with a six-day loading phase of creatine (0.3 grams per kilogram of body weight per day) and then initiated caffeine supplementation following the loading period and found greater exercise time to exhaustion and oxygen consumption. Therefore, it is difficult to state with certainty that caffeine negatively influences creatine ergogenicity, because caffeine itself is ergogenic and can improve athletic performance.

Supplementation Strategies

Creatine supplementation strategies must consider how rapidly muscle creatine content can be maximized, how well elevated muscle levels of creatine can be maintained, the timing of supplementation, and how long creatine levels can be elevated upon disuse (i.e., between cycles). Studies show that inclusion of the typical creatine loading phase (e.g., 20 to 30 grams of creatine, four or five times per day for five to seven days) maximizes muscle creatine content within a few days. Typically, a maintenance phase follows, consisting of 2 to 5 grams of creatine per day (or 0.03 grams per kilograms of body mass per day) for as long as the cycle lasts. Studies show that this dose is effective for maintaining creatine content. A key question athletes and coaches have is whether it is necessary to include a loading phase to receive maximal benefits. The answer is no, a loading phase is not necessary. However, attaining the peak level of creatine content will take longer if the loading phase is not included, but the end point will be the same. In addition, after loading with creatine, muscle creatine content remains elevated beyond the presupplementation period of approximately four to seven weeks (known as a "washout" period).

This information is important for athletes who cycle creatine because it can help in developing proper "off" cycling periods. Note that the cycling of creatine has not been studied in athletic populations. Cycling is important because it may create a greater potential for long-term progression and perhaps reduce the chance of creatine "abuse" taking place. Because muscle creatine levels plateau in a short period time, many experts suggest that most of the ergogenic effects of creatine supplementation take place early, which would mean that cycling may be useful for more long-term adaptations. Although not adequately studied at this point, one potential strategy is to load for one week, maintain for several weeks (e.g., eight to 12), reduce intake until complete disuse for up to six weeks, and then repeat the cycle (with the loading phase being optional; the athlete could simply initiate the next cycle with a maintenance dose). It appears that the timing of consumption (i.e., either before or after the workout/practice session) is not critical to performance enhancement because once peak muscle creatine content is achieved, subsequent performance should theoretically be equivalent. Some athletes prefer supplementing prior to a workout with the belief that more energy will be available for a more intense session, while others prefer postexercise supplementation to enhance the recovery process. Clearly, timing is not an issue during a loading phase, but it is during a maintenance phase if the athlete takes the supplement in one daily dose. These two timing options appear equally effective in the enhancement of athletic performance.

Types of Creatine Supplements

Many creatine supplements are available on the market. The most commonly used supplement among athletes is the powder form of *creatine monohydrate*, which can be mixed with water or any beverage containing sugar. *Creatine phosphate* and *creatine citrate* are also available. However, each of these forms contains less creatine per serving than creatine monohydrate.

Creatine, in general, comes in many forms, including capsules, gum, and liquid. The evolution of different forms stems from companies attempting to increase the rate of absorption, minimize gastric distress and bloating, and minimize residue when mixed. For example, micronized creatine reduces the size of creatine mixed and is thought to increase the rate of absorption and lessen residue. Also, effervescent creatine is thought to reduce bloating and increase absorption. Does a difference exist in the efficacy of these variants? The answer is no. Perhaps some forms (e.g., micronized, effervescent) may be absorbed faster, but the end point (i.e., the amount stored in the muscle) is the same. The stored amount within muscle is what provides energy for strenuous workouts and tough practices. Therefore, many forms of creatine are equally effective, though creatine monohydrate is very popular from a cost perspective. Lastly, creatine ethyl ester products are now available. The ester is attached to creatine to increase uptake to a greater extent. To date, no studies have compared the responses of supplementing with creatine ester to other creatine mixtures.

It is important to note that creatine comes in multipurpose supplements as well. For example, creatine is added to protein powders, glutamine, weight gainers, and other popular supplements to provide more ergogenicity. What does science have to say about these different creatine supplements? Consuming creatine with carbohydrates certainly has the most impact and is the only supplemental form shown to increase muscular creatine content more than just consuming creatine with water. Other studies have shown that creatine monohydrate, creatine candy, and creatine phosphate produced similar increases in muscular strength. More recently, it was shown that creatine and a creatine-magnesium chelated supplement (i.e., magnesium bound to creatine to reduce gastric breakdown) produced similar increases in performance, and creatine monohydrate was more effective for increasing sprint performance than creatine serum (Selsby et al., 2004; Gill et al., 2004).

Changes in Body Composition

Body composition includes an athlete's body weight, percent body fat, and lean tissue mass. Most studies have shown that creatine supplementation significantly increases body mass. As mentioned previously, most of the initial weight gain is in the form of water retention. However, this water retention is an osmotic signal to the body to increase muscle hypertrophy. Therefore, the initial water weight gain eventually becomes muscle mass. In fact, the range of increases in body mass reported in the literature is 0.6 to 5.2 kilograms for short- and long-term studies. These increases take place within the first seven days of supplementation, and some further increases may take place during longer supplementation periods. The increases in body mass are more prominent in male athletes, but women also tend to respond well to creatine supplementation.

As body mass increases, lean-tissue mass increases as well, mostly in the form of muscle mass. This effect is desirable for many anaerobic sports such as football, weight lifting, and track and field (throwing events). However, weight gain is not desirable in ultraendurance sports or in sports in which weight classes are used. The added weight gain could potentially hinder performance. For example, a high jumper or gymnast would have to produce more muscular force and power to overcome the additional weight. An endurance athlete would have to perform with additional weight for an extended period time. If the performance enhancement outweighs the weight gain, then creatine supplementation could be advantageous. Coaches and athletes need to recognize the importance of body-weight gain when considering supplementing with creatine.

Creatine supplementation may either reduce or have no affect on percent body fat. It is important to note that fat mass typically remains the same. However, an increase in lean tissue mass reduces percent body fat.

Performance Enhancement

The majority of studies have shown that creatine enhances performance, especially in anaerobic-type events (Figure 6-4). Several health- (i.e., strength, endurance) and skill-related components (i.e., power, speed, agility) of fitness have been improved in various studies. Although only some measures of sport-specific performance have been assessed, it is believed that the improvements in strength and power will translate into greater performances on the athletic field. Though difficult to measure directly, creatine supplementation does appear to enhance several aspects of performance, especially among athletes involved in anaerobic sports.

Rawson and Volek (2003) examined 22 studies that investigated creatine's effect on muscular strength and reported the average maximal strength increases was 8 percent and the average improvement in lifting performance (i.e., repetitions performed in the workout) was 14 percent greater than when supplementing with a placebo. The range of bench press improvements was 3 to 45 percent. Similar results have been obtained when examining various facets of muscular power. In our study

- Isometric strength and endurance
- Maximal grip strength
- 1-RM strength
  - ✓ Bench press
  - ✓ Squat
  - ✓ Power clean
  - ✓ Arm curl
  - ✓ Leg press
- Maximal repetitions to fatigue
- Isokinetic strength
- Ballistic power
  - ✓ Jump squat
  - ✓ Bench press throw
- Vertical jump height and power
- Strength and power maintenance during overreaching
- Sprinting speed
- Mean and peak cycling power
- Swimming sprint performance
- Agility
- Skating speed
- Soccer dribbling speed
- Kayaking performance

Figure 6-4. Performance enhancement with creatine supplementation

(Volek et al., 2004), creatine supplementation was effective for maintaining performance during high-volume overreaching, which resulted in strength and power reductions when supplementing with a placebo. The creatine-supplemented group enhanced their strength and power to a greater extent after the initial stress of overreaching. Although several studies have found no ergogenic potential with creatine supplementation, the majority of studies have indicated a strong potential for creatine to enhance athletic performance.

Another topic of interest is the effect of creatine supplementation on aerobic endurance. The question of whether aerobic athletes should supplement with creatine is frequently asked. The answer may depend on the duration and intensity of the sport. For example, some studies have shown that creatine supplementation can enhance performance of high-intensity aerobic events such as activities in which short bouts of exercise are followed by a recovery period, or increase the overall distance covered (e.g., during running) in the same or less time. Other studies have not duplicated those findings. It is important to note that these events include a strong anaerobic component as well and it is likely that creatine supplementation enhanced the anaerobic components that lead to enhanced performance during these short-to-moderate endurance events. Therefore, performance of relatively short interval events may be enhanced by creatine supplementation.

High- or ultra-endurance events have been studied less often, but they appear not to be enhanced by creatine supplementation. In fact, endurance athletes competing in these events need to keep their weight down and the potential weight gain from creatine supplementation may hurt performance to some extent. Therefore, high-duration, moderate-intensity aerobic athletes may not benefit sufficiently to warrant supplementation.

Why Don't Some Athletes Respond to Creatine Supplementation?

Some athletes do not benefit much from creatine supplementation. It has been estimated that 20 to 30 percent of subjects in creatine-supplementation studies were considered nonresponders because they experienced less than an 8 percent increase in total muscle creatine stores during loading (compared to the approximately 20 percent typically seen). Syrotuik and Bell (2004) examined profiles of "responders" and compared them to "nonresponders" and found that those individuals most responsive to creatine supplementation had lower levels of muscle creatine prior to supplementation, a substantial percentage of fast-twitch fibers, and a significant muscle size prior to supplementation. Responders also appear to gain strength significantly following only a five-day loading phase. Incidentally, this "responder" prototype is also indicative of athletes who excel in strength and power activities. Therefore, it is clear that some athletes will respond more favorably than others. However, even a slight increase in muscle creatine content could lead to better athletic performance.

Side Effects and Safety of Creatine Supplementation

Of major concern to a coach or athlete contemplating creatine supplementation are the potential side effects. Because of creatine's function as an osmotic agent, the potential for dehydration (and subsequent effects such as cramping) has been suggested, especially during exercise/competition in hot, humid environments. In addition, because excess creatine is metabolized to creatinine in the kidneys, potential overuse damage to the kidneys has also been suggested. Other organ (i.e., liver) damage has also been postulated. It is important to note that these concerns have primarily been raised via anecdotal sources such as newspapers, magazines, and the media in general.

In contrast to these reports, numerous studies have shown that creatine use is safe and that short-term creatine use has shown no negative impact on the kidneys or liver. Studies have shown that body temperature, blood pressure, and heart rate are not excessively elevated during exercise in the heat during creatine supplementation beyond the normal rise associated with exercise, and a study by Kilduff et al. (2004)

showed that the cardiovascular and thermoregulatory responses to exercise to exhaustion in the heat were lower in endurance athletes who supplemented with creatine. It is important to note that while creatine "use" appears safe, creatine "abuse" is a different matter. Creatine abuse is defined as long-term, excessive consumption of creatine. Consuming high doses for several weeks, months, or longer could potentially pose a problem to an athlete. Some athletes mistakenly believe that if "X" amount of a supplement works, then more than "X" should produce greater results. This expectation is unfounded and the additional supplementation may pose a health risk. Although science has not identified the long-term side effects (i.e., more than eight to 10 years), if any, that may develop via creatine supplementation, it is clear that short- to moderate-term usage is safe. It is also important that coaches and athletes understand that creatine supplementation has extended beyond the athletic realm and is now commonly used and studied in clinical populations, where its medical benefits are currently being identified.

- Reduction in the body's ability to synthesize creatine
- Increased urinary creatinine excretion, especially during loading phases
- Increased gastrointestinal distress (cramping)
- Dehydration

To date, evidence does not support the contention that creatine supplementation either increases renal stress or results in changes in markers of muscle and liver damage, electrolytes, blood volume or blood pressure, or thermoregulatory function.

Figure 6-5. Health ramifications and known side effects of creatine supplementation

Minor side effects of creatine supplementation have been noted in some individuals. For example, a few reports have been made of gastrointestinal distress (e.g., upset stomach, diarrhea, vomiting), especially during creatine-loading periods. In some individuals, supplementation may be overwhelming at first, as the high osmotic load may have some adverse effects. Again, only minor side effects have been reported, and in only a few individuals. These effects are not the norm among the majority of users. Receiving greater attention in the media is the potential effect of creatine supplementation on the incidence of muscle cramps. Some episodes of cramping have been reported, but, in reality, it is hard to identify if creatine supplementation caused the cramps or if the cramps were merely the result of a combination of other factors such as temperature, humidity, dietary deficiencies, and/or the intensity and volume of exercise. Nevertheless, fluid intake should be increased when supplementing with creatine. If an athlete is training and competing in a hot/humid environment, fluid intake should be greater.

Injuries to Athletes

Another prevailing misconception is that creatine supplementation causes a larger number of injuries to athletes. This effect has typically been ascribed to a greater incidence of muscle cramps and, perhaps, tighter muscles, which could easily result in strains. Greenwood and colleagues (2003) found that the incidence of cramping, muscle tightness, strains, illness, and missed practices were either the same or lower among football players supplementing with creatine. In addition, Watsford and colleagues (2003) found that creatine supplementation did not increase muscle stiffness. The results of these studies show that creatine supplementation does not increase the incidence of injuries in athletes. The information currently circulating through the media is anecdotal and not based on scientific evidence.

Coaching Points

- Athletes in predominantly anaerobic sports can benefit from creatine supplementation, which is ergogenic.
- Although many creatine supplements exist, they all provide similar ergogenic effects.
- Creatine supplementation increases muscle creatine content and the effect is greater when carbohydrates are consumed simultaneously.

7

Prohormones

A prohormone is a molecule that is eventually converted into a more potent, active form of a hormone. From a sports-supplement perspective, the most sought-after prohormones are those that have the potential to be converted into the hormone *testosterone*, which is a powerful anabolic hormone that can significantly increase an athlete's muscle size, strength, power, and endurance. However, it is illegal to consume testosterone and other anabolic steroids without a medical purpose (although these drugs are commonly used illegally by athletes and other individuals striving to increase muscle mass and strength).

Considering the illegality of these hormonal drugs, other attempts have been made to increase the body's own levels of testosterone. Exercise itself, particularly resistance exercise, can increase blood concentrations of testosterone during, and immediately following, a workout. Another potential method is to supplement with prohormones to increase testosterone concentrations. Since the inception of the 1994 Dietary Supplement Health and Education Act (DSHEA), prohormones have been a popular over-the-counter nutrition supplement. One prohormone, androstenedione, was first used in the 1970s as a nasal spray by East German Olympic athletes. Prohormone supplementation has received national media attention over the past five to 10 years, and sales have skyrocketed, especially since the revelation that many prominent professional baseball players (and other athletes) were using them. However, their efficacy and legality have been questioned.

Testosterone Precursors: The Pathway to Testosterone?

Testosterone is synthesized from cholesterol in several steps (Figure 7-1) and intermediate compounds are formed along the pathway to synthesis. Several of these intermediates have found their way into the supplement industry. The most common testosterone precursors used for supplementation are dehydroepiandrosterone (DHEA), 4-androstenediol, 5-androstenediol, and androstenedione, and 19-norandrostenediol and 19-norandrostenedione, which are nortestosterone (i.e., a potent steroid very similar to testosterone) precursors.

Theoretically, the fewer the number of conversion steps, the greater the likelihood of testosterone synthesis. In other words, those intermediates further along the reaction chain to testosterone are thought to more readily convert to testosterone, leading to transient elevations. This claim is made by many supplement manufacturers. It is thought that androstenediol conversion to testosterone is more efficient in the delta 4 pathway. Therefore, 4-androstenediol supplements are popular. It is also thought that androstenediol is three times more readily convertible to testosterone than androstenedione. However, the results from oral prohormone supplement studies have not shown much promise for either form. In addition, nortestosterone (e.g., nandrolone) is more potent and less androgenic than testosterone itself, because it has

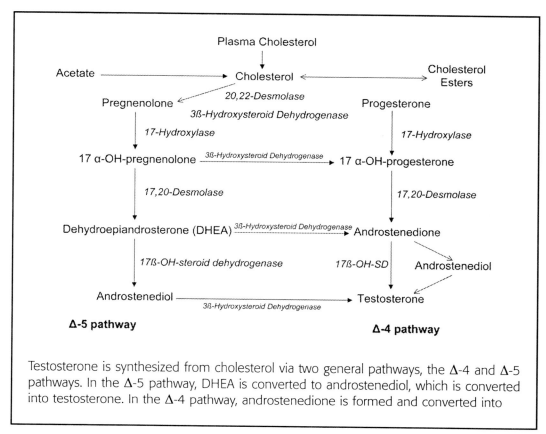

Testosterone is synthesized from cholesterol via two general pathways, the Δ-4 and Δ-5 pathways. In the Δ-5 pathway, DHEA is converted to androstenediol, which is converted into testosterone. In the Δ-4 pathway, androstenedione is formed and converted into

Figure 7-1. The pathway of testosterone synthesis

the nineteenth carbon removed. These factors have prompted athletes to use these precursor supplements due to greater proposed benefits and fewer side effects associated with higher estrogen levels. Norandrostenedione and norandrostenediol prohormone supplements (collectively called norandro supplements) are thought to synthesize into nortestosterone. However, research has shown that their ability to convert to the potent nortestosterone is also limited. Consequently, ergogenic potential is minimal without conversion.

General Actions of Prohormones

Prohormones, or testosterone precursors, basically perform the same functions as testosterone, but with far less potency. For the athlete, testosterone can:

- Increase muscle and bone mass
- Decrease body fat
- Increase muscle strength, power, and endurance
- Increase the ability to recover between workouts and competitions
- Increase blood volume
- Increase aggression

The critical information that you and your athletes need to know is that a conversion to testosterone must take place for these supplements to be effective. DHEA, androstenedione, and androstenediol are relatively weak androgens and they are very limited in performance. The reason for the ineffectiveness is their limited ability to interact with the androgen receptor. When androgens are released into circulation, they travel through the blood (with a transporter) to the target tissues (e.g., muscle, bone). Because andro and DHEA supplements are steroid hormones, they diffuse through the membrane and bind to the *androgen receptor*, which initiates the events leading to the aforementioned actions. Therefore, an androgen's potency is determined by its half-life and its binding, affinity, and interaction with the androgen receptor. Testosterone binds with greater affinity and stability to the androgen receptor, and its actions are therefore long-lasting and very potent. The andros and DHEA bind very weakly. Therefore the subsequent actions are limited. As a result, in their current form these prohormones have very little (if any) effect on athletic performance.

The Acute Response to Prohormone Supplements: Do They Increase Testosterone Levels?

The initial study that suggested prohormones may naturally increase testosterone was conducted by Mahesh and Greenblatt in 1962. Only two women were examined in this study, but a greater than 300 percent increase in testosterone was observed one hour after the ingestion of 100 milligrams of androstenedione. Several criticisms can be made about this study, but the premise for prohormone supplementation was established. Since the late 1990s, several acute-response studies have been conducted (Figure 7-2).

Collectively, these studies show dramatic increases in blood concentrations of DHEA and androstenedione. However, very little conversion to testosterone or the biologically active free testosterone took place. Only five of these studies showed an elevation and the supplemental dose used in these studies was higher than the recommended amount of 100 milligrams, and the response was more prominent in women. Why didn't testosterone levels increase consistently in these studies? It is possible that relatively low supplemental doses were used (compared to what athletes typically consume). In addition, in most cases, young, healthy men were studied (who already have high levels of testosterone). Therefore, an increase in testosterone levels would be less likely. Finally, the timing of the measurements may not have corresponded to peak hormonal values. Collectively, the answers to this question deal with metabolism of the prohormones. Oral prohormone use has limitations related to metabolism once ingested. In any case, the ultimate question is whether these supplements increase athletic performance.

Prohormone Supplementation and Performance Enhancement: Does a Link Exist?

Several studies have examined chronic oral prohormone supplementation over eight to 12 weeks during resistance training. These studies have unanimously shown that no additional increases in muscular strength and lean body mass took place. In addition, supplementation with norandrostenedione and norandrostenediol supplements had no ergogenic effects. Based on the doses and designs used in these studies, the data indicate that oral prohormone supplementation (whether testosterone levels increase or not) does not have a chronic ergogenic effect on performance.

Reference	Subjects	Treatment	Results
Labrie et al., 1997	Adult men/women	10 ml DHEA/day for two weeks	↑ DHEA, DHEA-S, and andro ↔ T, DHT, estrogens
Leder et al., 2000	Adult men	Androstenedione 7 days, 100 vs. 300 mg/day	**↑ T (300 mg only)** ↑ estrogens
Earnest et al., 2000	Adult men	200 mg of 4-androstene-3, 17-dione vs. 4-androstene-3ß, 17ß-diol	**↑ T, FT,** ↔ delta 4-diol
King et al., 1999	Young men	100 mg (acute response) and 300 mg/day for eight weeks of RT	↔ T, FT, ↓HDL ↑ estradiol, estrone
Ballantyne et al., 2000	Adult men	200 mg androstenedione	2- to 3-times ↑ androstenedione ↑70% LH and estradiol (83%), ↔ T
Wallace et al., 1999	Middle-aged men	100 mg/day DHEA or androstenedione for 12 weeks	↑DHEA-S ↔ blood lipids
Brown et al., 1999	Young men	50 mg DHEA	150% ↑ androstenedione ↔ LH, T, FT
Leder et al., 2000	Adult men	Androstenedione for 7 days, 100 vs 300 mg/day	**↑ T (300 mg only)** ↑ estrogens
Brown et al., 2000	Middle-aged men	Androstenedione 300 mg/day for 28 days	↑andro (300%), **FT (45%)**, DHT (83%), estradiol (68%) ↔ T, ↓HDL (10%)
Beckham & Earnest 2003	Middle-aged men	Androstenedione 200 mg/day for 28 days	↑andro ↔ T, blood lipids
Acacio et al., 2004	Adult men	50 or 200 mg/day DHEA for six months	↑ DHEA, DHEA-S ↔ T
Broeder et al., 2000	Middle-aged men	Androstenedione or androstenediol 200 mg/day for 12 weeks	↑ DHEA-S, androstenedione, estrone, estradiol ↔ T, FT, ↓HDL
Brown et al., 2001	Middle-aged men	Androstenediol 300 mg and herbs for 28 days	**↑ FT (37%)**, andro and (174%), DHT (57%), estradiol (86%) ↔ T, LDL, ↓HDL
Brown et al., 2004	Young women	Androstenedione 100 or 300 mg/day	**↑ T, estradiol**

Note: Boldface denotes an elevation in testosterone; DHEA-S = DHEA sulfate; DHT = dihydrotestosterone; ml = milliliters; mg = milligrams; ↑ = increase; ↓ = decrease; ↔ = no change; RT = resistance training; FT = free testosterone; T = testosterone; LH = luteinizing hormone

Figure 7-2. Acute response to prohormones

Metabolism of Prohormones

The key to the lack of significant results with oral prohormone use may relate to their metabolism. Leder and colleagues (2000) extensively examined oral androstenedione supplementation (100 and 300 milligrams) and found that urinary excretion rates of androgen metabolites increase in proportion to the amount of supplement consumed. They also found that prohormones do convert to testosterone, but predominantly in the liver, where 89 percent of the converted testosterone is excreted and does not reenter circulation. They also found that approximately 3 percent of androstenedione and approximately 15 percent of androstenediol may actually get converted to testosterone, but their data show that most of the testosterone is metabolized before traveling to specific target tissues. These results prove the minimal effectiveness of oral prohormone supplements.

What if prohormones were consumed in a different manner (other than orally)? This hypothesis was tested by Brown and colleagues in 2002. They studied the effects of 25 milligrams of sublingual (i.e., under the tongue) androstenediol and found substantial elevations in total and free testosterone. In other words, the metabolism appears to be the key issue. Oral prohormone supplements (at least in low-to-moderate doses) lose their efficacy, which may explain, in part, some of the poor results obtained with their use.

Prohormone Considerations: The Dreaded Side Effects

Prohormones produce some undesirable side effects that outweigh any potential benefits (and the benefits appear minimal at best). From a health standpoint, testosterone and its precursors are metabolized to *estrogens* (i.e., estradiol, estrone, estriol). In women, estrogens promote the development of female secondary sexual characteristics, such as breasts, and are also involved in controlling the menstrual cycle. In men, some side effects can occur when high levels of estrogens are present via aromitization from testosterone or its precursors. These side effects may include enlargement of the breast tissue (gynecomastia), female-pattern fat distribution, and water retention. Because of these effects, some athletes have used antiestrogens, which either block estrogens from binding to receptors or inhibit the aromatase enzyme to prevent estrogen formation. Several antiestrogens are prescription drugs. While some companies have marketed over-the-counter antiestrogens, their effects have not been tested (e.g., 6-Oxo from Ergopharm, Figure 7-3).

In addition, some masculinizing effects may take place with steroid use, especially in women. Men can also experience some problems associated with steroid use (e.g.,

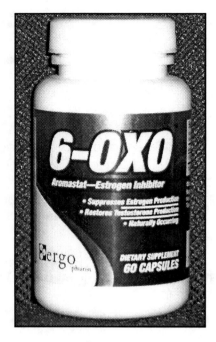

Figure 7-3. Over-the-counter anti-estrogen

decreased HDL, increased LDL). In addition, prohormone use can result in failed drug tests. Prohormones metabolize to common metabolites (e.g., 19-norandrosterone) similar to those of anabolic steroids (e.g., nandrolone) in a dose-dependent manner. Therefore, an athlete taking prohormone supplements can fail a drug test. A single dose of 50 milligrams may result in a failed test seven to 10 days later. Consuming 300 milligrams of androstenedione per day may result in slight elevations of the testosterone/epitestosterone ratio (i.e., T/E ratio, a marker used to detect testosterone use). Testosterone appears more quickly in the urine than epitestosterone does, so taking prohormones soon before a test could result in a T/E ratio of greater than 4:1, which is the criteria for a positive test.

The Crackdown on Andro Supplements

As part of a crackdown on andro supplements, the Food and Drug Administration (FDA) sent letters on March 11, 2004, to 23 companies, asking them to stop distributing supplements that contained androstenedione and warning them that they could face enforcement actions if they did not take appropriate action. The FDA announced that dietary supplements containing andro were adulterated ingredients under the DSHEA of 1994. A new dietary ingredient is defined as one that was not marketed in the United States before October 15, 1994. New dietary ingredients have to meet certain requirements, and because these requirements have not been met for androstenedione, supplements containing andro cannot be marketed legally. Therefore, DSHEA enabled the FDA to stop the sales of andro supplements. This action was taken due to concerns about safety issues related to andro products. Therefore, manufacturers and distributors ceased the selling of andro-related products, but not of DHEA. Stated simply, it is not recommended that andro supplements be taken by athletes.

Coaching Points

- Andro supplements are hormones that can result in a failed drug test.
- Most studies have failed to show any ergogenicity of andro supplements.
- Based on their recent ban and lack of efficacy, andro supplements are not recommended for athletes.

8

Sodium Bicarbonate and Sodium Citrate

Sodium bicarbonate (i.e., "baking soda") is an alkaline salt used to enhance performance. Its ergogenic potential was first observed in the 1920s. Research on *bicarbonate loading* was resurrected in the late 1970s, when studies were conducted examining the effects of higher doses. Sodium bicarbonate is the most commonly studied alkaline salt (other examples include sodium citrate and potassium bicarbonate). In contrast to many other supplements, numerous studies have been done examining exercise performance and supplementation with either sodium bicarbonate or citrate. The results have been somewhat controversial because many studies have shown performance enhancement, while several others have shown no additional improvement. This chapter focuses on the potential ergogenic benefits of sodium bicarbonate and citrate supplementation.

Rationale for Supplementation

High-intensity exercise leads to a rapid onset of fatigue. For exercise bouts lasting longer than 20 to 30 seconds, the breakdown of muscle glycogen (i.e., anaerobic glycolysis) becomes the major energy source. A by-product of anaerobic glycolysis is lactic acid, which, in part, is associated with several metabolic disturbances that lead to fatigue (*metabolic acidosis*). The amount of lactic acid produced ultimately depends upon the intensity and duration of exercise, as well as the training status of the athlete (i.e., much less lactic acid is produced in endurance-trained athletes than in sprint-trained athletes). The hydrogen ion (H^+) is critical to the onset of fatigue. Although the H^+ accumulates from other metabolic processes as well, H^+ dissociates from lactic acid (which becomes lactate) and lowers blood and muscle pH. The increase in H^+ (and decrease in pH) results in reduced muscle-force production and interferes with enzymes involved with energy production. Consequently, H^+ needs to be buffered to minimize the deleterious effects of fatigue.

The importance of pH homeostasis to sports performance cannot be overstated. The maintenance of acid-base balance is a collective effort among the pulmonary, renal, circulatory, and muscular systems, which work to buffer and excrete H^+ and remove excess carbon dioxide. The human body has several ways to buffer H^+ (e.g., phosphates, protein, carnosine). However, the bicarbonate system is of primary importance for enhancing buffer capacity. The bicarbonate anion (HCO_3) accepts H^+ to form carbonic acid (H_2CO_3), which is subsequently converted to water (H_2O) and carbon dioxide (CO_2). By buffering H^+ in the blood, a larger gradient is created between the muscle and extracellular H^+ concentrations that leads to an increase in H^+ efflux out of the muscle. The H^+ efflux out of muscle helps prolong high-intensity exercise performance.

Intake of sodium bicarbonate ($NaHCO_3$) results in an increase in blood pH and bicarbonate concentrations. It is thought that sodium bicarbonate supplementation may act to buffer the blood, thereby increasing the rate of H^+ efflux from muscle. In addition, because bicarbonate is a buffer, higher concentrations of H^+ can be produced and tolerated. In other words, although more H^+ is produced, it is buffered more efficiently, so it will not have the same impact in causing fatigue. With this rationale in mind, it is believed that supplementation with sodium bicarbonate can reduce fatigue and enhance performance in athletes.

Performance Enhancement

Studies examining bicarbonate loading have shown conflicting results. Some factors that have made it difficult to draw conclusions with certainty are the doses used, the timing of intake, the type of exercise protocol used, the amount of alkalosis gained through loading, and the training status of the subjects or athletes studied. Ultimately, the metabolic demands of the athletic event dictate the potential effects of bicarbonate loading. Because of its potential to buffer glycolytic by-products, the largest effects may be seen with high-intensity interval or anaerobic events. Some early studies showed that bicarbonate loading reduced 800-meter run times in middle-distance runners, increased time to exhaustion during cycling bouts, and resulted in faster 400-meter race times, higher power output during sprints, and greater interval swim performances. However, some studies using similar doses and protocols showed no ergogenic effects of sodium bicarbonate loading.

In addition, bicarbonate loading may or may not affect weight-training performance and does not increase $\dot{V}O_2$ max. In a meta-analysis, it was determined that the overall bicarbonate-loading effect was ergogenic (54 percent of studies showed substantial effects, while 46 percent showed little to no effect), with the largest effect seen when exercise protocols were performed to exhaustion. Interestingly, the studies that showed the largest ergogenic effects included subjects who experienced the largest amount of alkalosis (i.e., those who began with a somewhat low pH but had a substantial increase following loading). Therefore, performance enhancement was greatest when subjects were most responsive to the loading protocol.

Determining the type of activity that bicarbonate loading can best enhance is of obvious interest. It is thought that short, high-intensity exercise sessions lasting between one and seven minutes would yield performance improvement. For example, performance of interval training is thought to be enhanced because of its intense nature. In addition, higher blood-lactate levels could be achieved during the rest periods, and the efficacy of bicarbonate loading is greater as blood lactate levels increase. This fact was shown by McNaughton (1992b), who found that sodium bicarbonate loading enhanced performance during two- and four-minute exercise protocols, but did not affect 10- and 30-second protocols. Therefore, exercise sessions resulting in high levels of blood lactate may be most responsive to bicarbonate loading. Most studies have shown bicarbonate loading does not enhance aerobic-endurance performance. Strength and power athletes may not benefit from bicarbonate loading based on the duration and metabolic nature of these activities.

One less-studied factor is chronic supplementation with sodium bicarbonate. McNaughton and colleagues (1999) and McNaughton and Thompson (2001) provided subjects with 0.5 grams per kilogram of body mass per day of sodium bicarbonate over five and six days, respectively. Peak power during 60 seconds of high-intensity cycle exercise was enhanced during both protocols. However, more work was performed via supplementation over six days, and this effect was shown after the second day of loading. Ingestion over a period of days may also help relieve the gastrointestinal problems that can arise.

Supplement Doses and Timing

Another critical factor is how much sodium bicarbonate should be taken to increase athletic performance. Common doses have ranged from 100 to 500 milligrams per kilogram of body mass. Most studies have effectively used 300 milligrams per kilogram of body mass. However, for some interval protocols a dose of 200 milligrams per kilogram of body mass per day was found to be just as effective. McNaughton (1992a) compared bicarbonate loading with 100 to 500 milligrams per kilogram of body mass per day and found that doses of 200 to 500 milligrams per kilogram of body mass per day produced ergogenic effects, but 300 milligrams per kilogram of body mass per day was the most ergogenic dose for maximizing peak power.

The timing of supplementation is another factor to consider. Most studies have given the doses all at once or dispersed them over as long as a three-hour period. In addition, the range of time before the exercise session has ranged from immediately before to three hours prior to exercise. The majority of studies have loaded bicarbonate one to two hours before the exercise protocol was to begin. When 300 milligrams per kilogram of body mass per day is given, blood bicarbonate levels and pH increase within 20 to 30 minutes. However, peak values are seen approximately 90 to 120 minutes postingestion. Therefore, ingestion of sodium bicarbonate 90 to 120 minutes precompetition may be effective.

Side Effects

Bicarbonate loading is safe, but higher doses (greater than 300 milligrams per kilogram of body mass) may cause gastrointestinal (GI) distress (i.e., diarrhea, stomach upset/pain, cramping, vomiting). Most studies using higher doses have shown GI distress unless the doses are dispersed into smaller units. GI distress may be linked to the high sodium load involved, which can attract more water into the gut. Ingesting plenty of water during loading may relieve some or most of the distress.

Sodium Citrate Supplementation

Sodium citrate, after ingestion, is rapidly dissociated into sodium and citrate. Citrate is then expelled from the blood, which causes an electrical imbalance that results in alkalosis via an increase in bicarbonate or a reduction in H^+. Citrate plays important aerobic metabolic roles within muscle as well. Loading with sodium citrate can increase blood bicarbonate levels similar to, or even slightly more than, bicarbonate loading. As with bicarbonate loading, loading with sodium citrate may not improve performance of high-intensity activity lasting 10 to 30 seconds. However, exercise performance of bouts of 120 to 240 seconds can be enhanced. Sodium citrate loading (525 milligrams per kilogram of body mass) can increase maximal sprints, but is not quite as effective as sodium bicarbonate. Other studies showing the ergogenicity of sodium citrate (using 500 milligrams per kilogram of body mass) have shown greater improvements in 3,000-meter run times, 5-kilometer run times, and cycling time trials.

In trying to determine the optimal dose, McNaughton (1990) compared doses of 100 and 500 milligrams per kilogram of body mass per day and found that 500 milligrams produced the greatest increases in total work and peak power during one minute of cycling. However, some studies have shown no ergogenic effects with 300 to 500 milligrams per kilogram of body mass. It has been suggested that sodium citrate may cause less gastric distress than sodium bicarbonate, but some studies have shown similar low-distress responses to both sodium citrate and bicarbonate. Sodium citrate can be ergogenic when ingested 100 to 120 minutes before competition and at higher doses (500 milligrams per kilogram of body mass per day) than sodium bicarbonate. The combination of bicarbonate and citrate loading has been shown to produce similar, nonsignificant changes compared to either bicarbonate or citrate alone.

Ethics

Sodium bicarbonate and citrate loading is legal in sports, but some feel it may violate the International Olympic Committee's legislation concerning consumption of a substance in very large quantities to enhance sports performance. In addition, some athletes have used it to produce alkaline urine, which can mask drug tests (although pH may be checked during testing and an out-of-range pH may necessitate another sample). The ethics of these supplements can be debated from two view points. Some view it as similar to carbohydrate loading, in which a large dose is ingested to produce supercompensation. However, others view it as similar to blood doping, which is illegal. Nevertheless, urine testing is not feasible, as other substances can produce alkaline urine in addition to sodium bicarbonate or citrate. The ultimate decision of whether to bicarbonate load lies with coaches and athletes.

Coaching Points

- Sodium bicarbonate loading may be ergogenic for high-intensity exercise performance one to seven minutes in duration.

- An effective dose is 300 milligrams per kilogram of body mass taken 90 to 120 minutes before competition with plenty of fluids.

- Taking smaller doses in increments (as opposed to all at once) may help relieve potential gastrointestinal distress.

- Bicarbonate loading has minimal to no effect on enhancing strength or power events lasting less than 60 seconds (with long rest intervals in between) or low-intensity endurance training.

- Sodium citrate can be ergogenic when ingested 100 to 120 minutes before competition and at high doses (500 milligrams per kilogram of body mass per day).

- Coaches can experiment with loading during training or practice to introduce athletes to the mechanics of loading. Loading before an event for the first time can be very counterproductive if athletes are not used to potential side effects.

9

Herbal Supplements

Herbal supplements contain plants or plant extracts that include a variety of phytochemicals (e.g., plant sterols, saponins, flavonoids, sulfides, carotenoids phthalides, terpenoids, lignans, coumarins, and polyphenolics). In supplement form, herbal extracts are more desirable than the herbs themselves, as the extracts contain a higher proportion of the active ingredients. Many different herbs are used in supplement form, and some of the more commonly used examples typically claim that athletes will have greater levels of energy, strength, and power; higher testosterone concentrations; increased muscle mass, mental focus and weight loss; decreased body fat; and better general health (e.g., improved immune and cardiovascular function).

In the United States, most herbs fall within the realm of DSHEA, and therefore are typically found in many types of supplements (e.g., powders, bars, multipurpose supplements), as well as being available individually. Most of the supplements listed in Figure 9-1 have been shown to be safe for supplementation in healthy individuals or athletes when consumed in moderation. However, caution is necessary for some, such as ephedra, *citrus aurantium*, and caffeine, which could lead to positive urinary drug tests. Ephedra was once banned, though this ban has since been overturned. Although clinical research has been performed on several of these herbal supplements, very few studies have examined their ergogenic potential in athletes. Therefore, many of the purported effects have been suggested based on some remote physiological findings or anecdotal theories.

Ginseng

Ginseng is regularly supplemented by more than six million Americans, with annual sales exceeding $300 million. The term "ginseng" actually refers to panax ginseng, or

Herb	Reason for Use	Comments
Arctic rose (*rhodiola rosea*)	↑ energy and endurance, adaptogen*	200 mg ↑ time to exhaustion and $\dot{V}O_2$; 300 mg in a herbal supplement did not affect cycling performance **possibly ergogenic
Asian ginseng (*panax ginseng*)	↑ energy and endurance, ↓ blood pressure, ↑ memory, recovery, and immunity (adaptogen)	Conflicting reports between studies showing ergogenicity and those showing none **possibly ergogenic
B-sitosterol [and other sterols such as gamma oryzanol (GO)]	↑ testosterone, endorphins, and muscle growth	500 mg/day of GO for 9 weeks of RT did not ↑ testosterone, GH, strength, or vertical jump *not ergogenic
Bitter orange (*citrus aurantium*); synephrine	↑ thermogenesis, energy, and weight loss	Similar to caffeine, ephedrine **possibly ergogenic for weight loss
Caffeine (guarana, kola nut)	↑ energy and endurance, thermogenesis, metabolism, strength, power, weight loss, body-fat reductions, and mental focus	Thermogenic and can enhance performance **ergogenic
Cayenne pepper (*capsicum frutescens*)	Pain relief, weight loss, blood-sugar control	Antidiabetic effect *not ergogenic
Chinese ephedra (ma huang; *ephedra sinica*)	↑ energy and endurance, thermogenesis, metabolism, strength, power, weight loss, body-fat reductions, and mental focus	Thermogenic, but several safety hazards Most effective when stacked with caffeine **ergogenic but banned for athletes
Chrysin (*passiflora coerulea*)	↑ testosterone by inhibiting aromatase activity; block conversion into estrogen	May or may not ↑ testosterone or ↓ estrogens; when added to andro, did not enhance strength *not ergogenic
Cordyceps (*cordyceps sinensis*)	Adaptogen, ↑ energy	No effect on muscle endurance, tissue oxygenation, and performance (1000 to 3000 mg) in cyclists *not ergogenic
Cystoseira canariensis	Binds to and inhibits myostatin (↑ strength, size)	12 weeks of RT with 1200 mg/day did not ↑ strength and mass or ↓ myostatin *not ergogenic
Gingko biloba	Increased blood flow, better circulation, antioxidant, stress reduction, mental acuity	Limited effects on performance; helps with peripheral artery disease *not ergogenic in healthy individuals

Figure 9-1. Herbs commonly touted to enhance athletic performance

Herb	Reason for Use	Comments
Glucomannan (*amorphophallus konjac*)	Nondigestible CHO, fiber-like, appetite suppressant, weight loss	Possible weight loss **not ergogenic*
Gurmar (*gymnema sylvestre*)	Blood-sugar control, improves insulin effects	Antidiabetic **not ergogenic*
Hydroxy citric acid (*garcinia cambogia*)	Appetite suppression, fat loss, ↑endurance	Conflicting reports, as some studies show greater fat loss and endurance and some do not ****possibly ergogenic**
Puncture vine (*tribulus terrestris*)	↑ testosterone	Alone may not ↑testosterone, but in combo with prohormones may ↑ free testosterone; does not enhance strength/ ↑endurance with RT **not ergogenic*
Saw palmetto (*serenoa serrulata*)	Prostate health, testosterone-like effects	No evidence for anabolic actions **not ergogenic*
Sarsaparilla (*smilax officinalis*)	↑ testosterone	Does not ↑testosterone in humans **not ergogenic*
Siberian ginseng (*eleutherococcus senticosus*)	↑endurance, energy, and recovery	Conflicting reports between studies showing ergogenicity and those showing none ****possibly ergogenic**
St. John's Wort (*hypericum perforatum*)	Antidepressant; pain and inflammation relief	May help depression **not ergogenic*
Suma (*pfaffia paniculata*); Brazilian ginseng	↑ endurance and stress toleration	May ↑ testosterone in mice; no evidence in humans **not ergogenic*
Wild (Mexican) yam (*dioscorea villosa*)	↓ inflammation and fatigue	Similar to progesterone and may have estrogenic effects **not ergogenic*
Willow bark (*salix alba*)	Pain relief, reduced inflammation	Possible pain relief **not ergogenic*
Yohimbe (*pausinystalia yohimbe*)	↓ body fat, ↑ blood flow, aphrodisiac,↓ blood lipids	No anabolic or performance effects ****possibly ergogenic for weight loss**

Note: ↓ = decrease; ↑ = increase; mg = milligrams; CHO = carbohydrate; RT = resistance training; GH = growth hormone
* *adaptogen* = normalizes physical functioning

Figure 9-1. Herbs commonly touted to enhance athletic performance (cont.)

Chinese or Korean ginseng. Many types of ginseng exist, with the differences depending on the origin and root maturity, the parts of the root used, and the processing technique. Some other forms of ginseng include panax quinquefolium (American ginseng), white ginseng, panax japonicus (Japanese ginseng), panax notoginseng (Sanchi), and eleutherococcus senticosus (Siberian ginseng). Ginseng has been used for several thousand years to increase energy, enhance immunity, and prevent disease. Ginseng is known as an adaptogen, which is a substance that keeps the body healthy. In addition, ginseng is thought to reduce stress by minimizing the catabolic effects of the hormone cortisol.

Ginseng's purported role as an energy/endurance enhancer is the critical reason why many athletes choose it as a supplement. More than 40 studies have been published examining ginseng's role in exercise and mental performance. Some early studies showed a potential ergogenic effect on endurance. However, many of those studies have been criticized for methodological flaws and possible bias, especially some of the Siberian ginseng studies. Therefore, it is still difficult to determine if, in fact, ginseng supplementation did increase athletic performance. In a review of the literature, Bucci (2000) reported that 10 out of 15 studies showed ergogenicity. In those studies, 200 to 2,000 milligrams of Panax ginseng resulted in increases in aerobic capacity, exercise time to exhaustion, pulmonary function, and postexercise recovery, as well as reduced lactate. Note that three of these ergogenic studies were performed using endurance athletes.

McNaughton and colleagues (1989) reported 13 to 27 percent increases in muscle strength following six weeks of supplementing with 1000 milligrams of Chinese or Siberian ginseng. However, research has shown a range of supplement doses from 200 milligrams to relative doses of 8 to 16 milligrams per kilogram of body mass of *Panax ginseng* supplementation for one to eight weeks had no effect on exercise time to exhaustion, $\dot{V}O_2$ max, blood lactate during exercise, and pulmonary function. Siberian ginseng supplementation (one to eight weeks) has been shown to not induce further improvements in $\dot{V}O_2$ max, time to exhaustion, pulmonary function, or cycling time trials in athletes in most studies, although a few studies did show greater endurance. Liang et al. (2005) have shown one month of supplementation with 1,350 milligrams per day of *panax notoginseng* increased aerobic endurance.

Because of the disparity in research findings and some well-controlled studies showing limited effects, it is difficult to recommend ginseng supplementation for endurance athletes. Although ergogenic potential may be questionable (despite high praise from some endurance athletes), some evidence does show that ginseng can improve health, and from that standpoint supplementation may be attractive. Panax ginseng may limit the muscle damage associated with eccentric exercise, which adds a new dimension to the purported effect of enhanced recovery. For those athletes who wish to experiment, ginseng supplementation is safe when taken in moderation and perfectly legal. Most studies have used supplemental doses of 200 to 1000 milligrams per day. Long-term overuse could result in high blood pressure, sleep disorders, and nervousness and anxiety.

Ephedra

Chinese ephedra (i.e., ma huang, ephedra sinica) has been used for more than 5,000 years for treating respiratory problems and is commonly seen in pharmaceuticals such as bronchodilators (for asthma), antihistamines, decongestants, and weight-loss products. The active ingredients include ephedrine and its alkaloids (pseudoephedrine, norephedrine, norpseudoephedrine, methylephedrine, phenylpropanolamine, and methylpseudoephedrine). The ephedrine content of different plants depends on where the plant was grown, the growing conditions, and the harvest time. Ephedra-containing product sales escalated between 1999 and 2000, with an estimated several billion dollars in sales taking place during that period. More than 100 individuals sued makers of ephedra products for safety issues between 2000 and 2002. While ephedra has been shown to be effective for weight loss and performance enhancement, much controversy has centered on this supplemental compound, leading to a temporary sales ban as well as a ban from various competitive athletic organizations.

Ephedrine use is banned by the International Olympic Committee (IOC) and the National Collegiate Athletic Association (NCAA). Because ephedrine alkaloids are found in common cold medicines, athletes need to be aware that consumption of these products can result in a failed drug test, especially since some products contain higher quantities of ephedrine alkaloids than what is reported on the label. Use of over-the-counter decongestants containing phenylpropanolamine and pseudoephedrine for 36 hours may result in peak drug urine concentrations four hours following the last dose. Elevations can persist for up to 16 hours. Urine concentrations of greater than 10 milligrams per liter of ephedrine and greater than 25 milligrams per liter of pseudoephedrine are considered positive drug tests by most sport-governing bodies.

Typical doses (prior to the ban) included 25 milligrams per pill or capsule, with recommendations to not exceed 100 milligrams per day. Some athletes, though, have reported much higher doses, in addition to "stacking" ephedrine with caffeine and aspirin. Analysis of ephedrine-related supplements revealed that 31 percent contained more than 110 percent of the amount listed on the label. The incidence of ephedrine use has been high in bodybuilders, weight lifters, and gym members, and reports show that approximately 3.4 percent of NCAA athletes have used ephedrine-related substances.

Ephedrine is classified as a sympathomimetic drug because it stimulates the central nervous system. The effects of "adrenaline" are similar to the effects of ephedrine on the human body. Its actions are also similar to amphetamines. Therefore, ephedrine may increase alertness, reduce fatigue, and perpetuate adrenaline. It is also thermogenic, meaning that it increases body temperature and metabolism, thereby burning fat and facilitating weight loss. A meta-analysis (Shekelle et al., 2003) showed that ephedrine and its alkaloids result in significant weight loss. Ephedrine also acts as a bronchodilator (which is why it is given to asthma patients) and cardiovascular stimulant, and it may reduce appetite. Ephedrine absorption is faster in capsule form, greater when ingested with caffeine-related herbs, and slower when it comes from ma huang. However, other effects may occur, such as nervousness, anxiety, heart palpations, headaches, nausea, cardiomyopathy, high blood pressure, and, in some rare cases, stroke. Some of these effects may be exacerbated during exercise in hot, humid conditions. In addition, long-term use may cause the body to rely on supplementation and lose the ability to produce its own adrenaline.

Performance changes with ephedrine use are less clear. An initial dose of approximately 57 to 120 milligrams of pseudoephedrine may not enhance fatigue parameters, power output, force, cycling time to exhaustion, or $\dot{V}O_2$ max. In addition, a combination of 60 milligrams of pseudoephedrine and 25 milligrams of phenylpropanolamine (six doses over 36 hours) may not enhance endurance-running performance. However, 180 milligrams of pseudoephedrine (45 minutes before exercise) results in greater peak power during cycling and muscle strength (Gill et al., 2000).

It should be noted that pseudoephedrine is approximately two-and-a-half times less potent than ephedrine. Studies examining ephedrine supplementation alone (i.e., one milligram per kilogram of body mass) have only shown a limited ergogenic effect on performance. Most studies show acute ephedrine supplementation does not enhance performance, although some studies do show ergogenic effects (i.e., a reduction in 10-kilometer run times and improved weight-training performance). However, these results were from acute studies that only looked at initial performance changes. Chronic adaptations to supplementation were not investigated. Therefore, the effects of ephedrine as a training tool remain relatively unknown, although some athletes report strength and performance improvements.

Ephedrine supplementation is most effective when stacked with caffeine, but it also has been effectively stacked with aspirin, yohimbe, and theophylline (a substance from the same family as caffeine—methylxanthines—with similar functions to caffeine and ephedrine). It is thought that caffeine and aspirin synergy potentiate the effects of ephedrine. The combination of caffeine and ephedrine can result in increases blood pressure, heart rate, blood glucose, minute ventilation, insulin, free fatty acids in the blood, and lactate concentrations during exercise. The combination of caffeine (5 milligrams per kilogram of body mass) and ephedrine (1 milligram per kilogram of body mass) has been shown to result in greater increases in power output and time

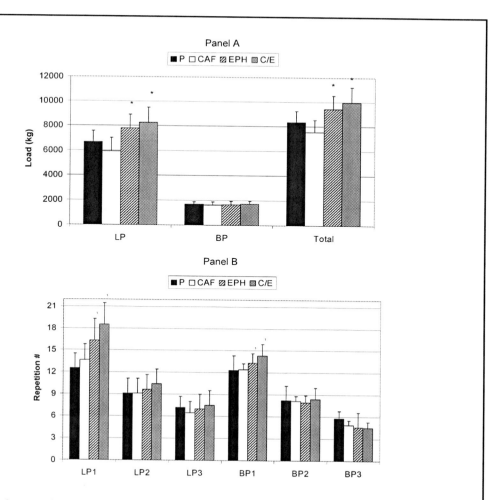

Panel A: Total work performed during three sets of strength training for the leg press (LP) and bench press (BP). Subjects either consumed a placebo (P), 4 milligrams per kilogram of body mass of caffeine (CAF), 0.8 milligrams per kilogram of body mass of ephedrine (EPH), or a combination of CAF and EPH (C/E). Consumption of EPH and C/E 90 minutes prior to exercise resulted in more work performed for LP and for total workload (LP + BP).

Panel B: Number of repetitions performed during three sets of LP and BP 90 minutes following supplementation. The results show that supplementation with EPH and C/E resulted in more repetitions performed during the first set of LP and BP. Overall, a 48 percent improvement in LP and a 16 percent improvement in BP occurred.

Figures modified from Jacobs and colleagues (2003).

Figure 9-2. The effects of caffeine, ephedrine, and a caffeine/ephedrine combination on acute lifting performance

to exhaustion during exercise 90 minutes following ingestion. Supplementation with 375 milligrams of caffeine and 75 milligrams of ephedrine can result in faster run times. In addition, a stack of caffeine (150 milligrams), aspirin (330 milligrams), and ephedrine (75 to 150 milligrams) is effective for weight loss in obese individuals. Caffeine/ephedrine stacking can enhance strength-training performance as well (Figure 9-2).

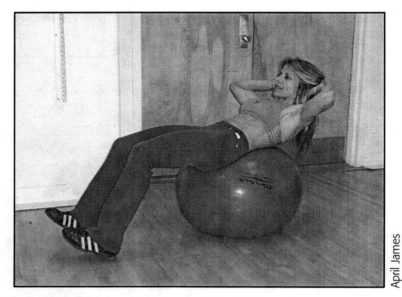

Figure 9-3. Athlete with low percent body fat

On February 6, 2004, the Food and Drug Administration (FDA) banned dietary supplements containing ephedrine alkaloids pending Congressional review. The ban culminated a seven-year regulatory process during which safety issues were of the utmost concern (ephedra was speculatively linked to more than 150 deaths). However, a federal judge on April 14, 2005, overturned the FDA's ban on ephedra. U.S. District Judge Tena Campbell in Salt Lake City characterized the FDA's ban as too broad, saying the agency did not demonstrate "a significant or unreasonable risk." Therefore, ephedra products are back on the shelves, although further challenges may be forthcoming.

Tribulus Terrestris

Tribulus terrestris (puncture vine) is an herbal preparation purported to increase testosterone concentrations and, subsequently, muscle strength and size. It has been used for many years (since the time of the Ancient Greeks) to improve sexual function in humans, reduce blood pressure and cholesterol, and treat headaches, nervous disorders, and constipation. It may also be a diuretic. The fruits of tribulus contain a number of different active substances, including saponins (protodioscin, furostanol). In animals, tribulus terrestris may increase testosterone via an increase in luteinizing hormone (LH), which is the hormone that actually causes testosterone secretion. However, the response in humans has been less dramatic.

Neychev and Mitev (2005) measured the response to 10 to 20 milligrams per kilogram of body mass of tribulus terrestris extract at 24, 72, 240, 408, and 576 hours postsupplementation. They did not find any differences in testosterone, LH, or androstenedione. The addition of tribulus terrestris (750 milligrams), as well as other herbals such as chrysin and saw palmetto, to andro supplements did not result in greater testosterone concentrations, strength increases, or lower estradiol. However, studies show that using a similar mixture did result in higher free testosterone levels in middle-aged men and a study (Brown et al., 2001) using another mixture (300 milligrams of androstenediol, 480 milligrams of saw palmetto, 450 milligrams of indole-3-carbinol, 300 milligrams of chrysin, 1,500 milligrams of gamma-linolenic acid, and 1,350 milligrams of tribulus terrestris) showed a 37-percent elevation in free testosterone, a 174-percent elevation in androstenedione, and an 86-percent elevation in estradiol in 30- to 58-year-old men over one month of supplementation. This study demonstrates that, when mixed with other supplements, tribulus may increase free testosterone. However, the logical question then is, "can it increase muscle strength and size over time?" Antonio and colleagues (2000b) examined supplementation with 3.2 milligrams per kilogram of body mass of tribulus for eight weeks during periodized strength training and found no further enhancement in maximal strength, muscle endurance, or body composition. Stated simply, no studies have shown an ergogenicity of tribulus supplementation.

Chrysin

Chrysin (a flavonoid) is a chemical extracted from the plant Passiflora coerulea. It is purported to elevate testosterone by inhibiting the enzyme aromatase, which converts testosterone into estrogens. By blocking this conversion, testosterone elevations should persist. Antiestrogens are particularly popular among anabolic steroid users in an effort to reduce some of the androgenic side effects. Therefore, chrysin, if effective, could serve multiple purposes. Although some evidence exists that flavonoids, especially chrysin, may reduce aromatase activity, its ergogenic potential on sports performance appears minimal. Consumption of foods high in chrysin [e.g., propolis ("bee glue"), honey] for 21 days was shown to not affect resting concentrations of testosterone. The addition of chrysin (625 milligrams), as well as other herbals such as tribulus terrestris and saw palmetto, to andro supplements does not result in greater testosterone concentrations, strength increases, or lower estradiol. However, a study using a similar mixture did show higher free testosterone in middle-aged men (Kohut et al., 2003). Not much conclusive evidence exists warranting the use of chrysin in an athlete's supplement regimen, at least not at the doses used in research.

Hydroxycitric Acid

Hydroxycitric acid (HCA) is derived from Garcinia cambogia and is purported to increase weight loss (mostly fat loss). HCA is an inhibitor of the enzyme citrate lyase (which is involved in lipid synthesis), and therefore it promotes fat oxidation (and appetite suppression) and is thought to lead to greater submaximal aerobic endurance. Studies have shown conflicting results. Some studies in obese subjects have shown low-dose supplementation with 750 milligrams to 3 grams per day of Garcinia cambogia or HCA reduces body weight, while several studies have not had the same results. A few studies have shown that 3 to 19 grams per day of HCA for up to three days before a standardized exercise protocol did not alter fat or carbohydrate metabolism but did slightly lower blood lactate. However, some studies have shown that 250 to 500 milligrams of HCA taken for five days increased fat oxidation, decreased carbohydrate oxidation, and enhanced exercise endurance in untrained individuals and athletes. Long-term exercise studies have not been performed, so HCA's effects on training adaptations are unknown. Conflicting reports make it difficult to recommend HCA supplementation, although higher doses appear to have a greater effect. HCA supplementation is legal and negative side effects have not been shown in these studies. However, because only short-term studies have been conducted, potential long-term side effects are still unknown.

Coaching Points

- Ginseng supplementation may improve general health, but the potential ergogenic effects are unknown.

- Many herbs are not ergogenic for enhancing performance. However, some may have health-promoting benefits.

- Several herbs (garcinia cambogia (HCA), ephedrine and ephedrine alkaloids, caffeine, yohimbe, glucomannan, bitter orange, cayenne pepper, and gurmar) are typically included in thermogenic supplements, because they either break down fat stores, decrease appetite, maintain or lower blood sugar levels (and insulin), and increase fat oxidation.

- For performance enhancement, caffeine, ephedrine, and stacks of both or in combination with aspirin or yohimbe, can increase muscular endurance, oxygen consumption, and race times. These herbs are the only ones to consistently show ergogenicity.

- Ephedra and related products were temporarily banned due to purported health risks. This ban has since been overturned. However, athletes can test positive and fail a drug test when ingesting ephedrine supplements within a few days of testing.

- Purported testosterone enhancers (i.e., sterols, chrysin, tribulus terrestris, saw palmetto, and smilax) have not been shown to increase testosterone or muscle mass unless stacked with prohormones.

10

Other Popular Sports Supplements

Many other sports supplements are commonly used by athletes but have not been discussed thus far in the book. This chapter focuses on several supplements, many of which have at least some slight ergogenic potential. Many of these supplements are amino acid derivatives. Supplements covered include acetyl and L-carnitine, arginine α-ketoglutarate ("nitric oxide" boosters), α-ketoisocaproate and β-HMB, β-alanine and carnosine, citrulline malate, cortitrol, glucosamine-chondroitin and hyaluronic acid, glutamine, ornithine α-ketoglutarate, octacosanol, pyruvate, and ribose.

Acetyl and L-Carnitine

Acetyl L-carnitine is composed of L-carnitine and acetic acid and is a more bioavailable form of L-carnitine. It facilitates the synthesis and release of the neurotransmitter acetylcholine, which is why it is used to treat various neurological disorders. Acetyl L-carnitine facilitates fat transport and oxidation. Some acetyl L-carnitine supplements contain *alpha lipoic acid*, an antioxidant that also helps carbohydrate metabolism. This combination is used because some studies have shown that with aging, fat-oxidation ability declines, with free radical damage and a reduction in carnitine levels possible factors. Therefore, acetyl L-carnitine-plus-alpha-lipoic-acid may restore carnitine levels and improve fat metabolism with aging. A study in rats (Bidzinska et al., 1993) showed that acetyl L-carnitine helped maintain testosterone levels during stressful swimming. However, no anabolic effects are evident in humans. Acetyl L-carnitine is typically sold in 500-milligram capsules and taken one to three times per day. From an ergogenic standpoint, no evidence supports that it can increase athletic performance.

L-carnitine is a compound that is synthesized from the amino acids lysine and methionine. Skeletal muscle is the main storage site for L-carnitine. It can be synthesized in the body (i.e., liver, kidneys) and humans get L-carnitine from dietary sources such as meat and dairy products. L-carnitine assists in transporting long-chain fatty acids across the inner membrane of the mitochondria, which is the part of the cell where aerobic energy metabolism takes place. Therefore, without L-carnitine a person's fat-burning capacity would be severely limited. In this fat-burning process, L-carnitine maintains appropriate levels of a molecule called acetyl CoA [and coenzyme A (CoA)]. Simply stated, if an appropriate ratio of these compounds is maintained, less lactic acid will be produced during moderate-to-high intensity exercise. L-carnitine increases fat metabolism, spares muscle glycogen, and can reduce lactic-acid formation during exercise. In addition, supplemental carnitine could potentially replace carnitine lost during exercise.

From a supplementation standpoint, L-carnitine has been touted as a "fat burner" and endurance enhancer. However, the key aspect of a potential ergogenic effect is that supplementation must increase the amount of L-carnitine in the muscles. Oral carnitine supplementation has been shown to have 5- to 15-percent bioavailability, meaning that only a small portion has the potential to be transported into skeletal muscle, while the majority is excreted in urine. Because total-body carnitine content is approximately 20 grams and bioavailability is low, L-carnitine supplemental doses are typically high in an attempt to produce some type of increase in muscle content. Also, Millington and Dubag (1993) have shown that many over-the-counter carnitine supplements contain far less carnitine than the labels state (approximately 52 percent less). Most studies show that supplementation does not increase muscle carnitine levels (with 4 to 5 grams per day of L-carnitine), despite large increases in blood carnitine concentrations.

Despite a lack of consistent findings of greater muscle content with L-carnitine supplementation, some studies have found ergogenic effects. In a few extensive reviews, 18 studies using L-carnitine supplementation of 1 to 6 grams per day for up to six weeks were reviewed. Of these 18 studies, 13 found no ergogenic effects of L-carnitine supplementation. Of the five studies showing ergogenicity, three found increases in $\dot{V}O_2$ max, three found reduced levels of lactic acid during exercise, and three found lower respiratory quotients (RQ; a measure of fuel source) during exercise, indicating greater use of fats as fuel. Most studies show limited ergogenic potential with L-carnitine supplementation, indicating that the body's own production level is sufficient to tolerate the exercise stress.

One follow-up question is obvious: If muscle content does not increase, then why did some studies find ergogenic changes? Some evidence exists that L-carnitine may perform some of its functions via other mechanisms. For example, some evidence shows that L-carnitine supplementation may alter hormonal responses favoring fat breakdown and oxidation. In fact, our research identified a different ergogenic effect. We found that carnitine supplementation (2 grams per day of L-carnitine L-tartrate for three weeks) improved blood flow and the delivery of oxygen to muscle tissue during and after resistance exercise, thereby reducing free radical–induced muscle damage and soreness by approximately 45 percent. No side effects were found, showing that L-carnitine supplementation is safe. L-carnitine supplementation (typically 2 to 5 grams per day) is legal and may be effective under certain conditions (e.g., recovery enhancement), although its fat-burning and endurance-enhancing effects are still debatable.

Arginine Alpha-Ketoglutarate and Nitric Oxide Boosters

Arginine alpha-ketoglutarate (A-AKG) is a salt formed by the combination of the amino acid arginine and a molecule of alpha-ketoglutarate (AKG). Because AKG is a metabolic intermediate and is involved in amino-acid synthesis (i.e., glutamine, glutamate, proline, arginine), many athletes use AKG supplements with hope of increasing muscle mass and strength via anticatabolic effects that reduce muscle breakdown, as AKG has been used in burn/trauma patients and to treat malnutrition. In addition, AKG may have a slight role in promoting a hormonal (insulin, growth hormone, IGF-1) response and wound healing. However, no evidence exists showing that strength/power athletes using AKG supplementation can enhance their muscle strength, size, and power. In fact, no studies have been conducted with athletes examining ergogenicity.

AKG supplements have experienced a surge in popularity, because A-AKG has the amino acid arginine bound within its complex. Arginine is a precursor to nitric oxide (NO), in which NO is formed via enzyme (nitric oxidase) activity. NO is a free form gas produced in the body that communicates with other cells and performs numerous relevant functions. For example, NO causes vasodilation (i.e., an increase in blood-vessel expansion), which leads to increased oxygen transport, blood flow, and nutrient delivery, and reduces blood pressure. A-AKG and arginine-alpha ketoisocaproate are common compounds found in NO supplements, as they increase NO concentrations. Exercise increases vasodilation and the addition of arginine results in an even greater magnitude of vasodilation. This effect potentially could have significant ramifications on training. Nitric oxidase activity is increased with training, and allowing more blood flow theoretically can result in greater strength and endurance. In fact, this enzyme is increased in response to strength training and may mediate some increases in muscle mass. High-volume, short-rest lifting sessions that result in high muscle blood flow and an accumulation of metabolites (i.e., "muscle pump") may be a potent stimulus for NO production. Therefore, NO supplements are very common among bodybuilders.

Nitric oxide supplements come in various forms. Many contain approximately three grams of arginine (A-AKG, arginine alpha-ketoisocaproate, and diarginine malate). In addition, multipurpose supplements are available to enhance workout/sports performance (e.g., creatine, nitric oxide supplements). No studies have been conducted looking at NO supplements and athletic performance. However, physiologically, NO does have ergogenic potential. Several studies will probably be completed in the next few years. Until then, recommendations state that supplementing with 3 grams of NO enhancers prior to a workout or competition may be beneficial.

Alpha-Ketoisocaproate and ß-HMB

Alpha-ketoisocaproate (KIC) is a keto acid of the branched-chain amino acid leucine. KIC is anticatabolic and has a protein-sparing effect. However, little evidence exists to show that supplementation with KIC is ergogenic. The ergogenic potential of KIC was identified when it was discovered that KIC had a more potent downstream compound in its pathway called β-*hydroxy-β-methylbutyrate* (HMB). Although it was thought that high amounts of KIC could increase protein synthesis, this effect has never been conclusively shown. However, the downstream metabolite HMB has received more attention and has been a very popular sports supplement.

Pathway: Leucine → KIC → HMB

Research has shown that many of the anabolic properties of leucine or KIC are due to its conversion to a more active form, HMB. A landmark study in this area was conducted by Nissen and colleagues (1996). They gave subjects a placebo, 1.5 grams of HMB per day, or 3.0 grams of HMB per day. The subjects were categorized based on protein intake and underwent three weeks of strength training three days per week. In addition, another group of subjects trained six days per week for seven weeks and were given either a placebo or 3.0 grams of HMB per day. Collectively, subjects who consumed 3.0 grams of HMB per day increased lean-tissue mass by 1.2 kilograms, while the control group (no HMB) increased lean-tissue mass by 0.4 kilograms and the group that consumed 1.5 grams of HMB saw a 0.8-kilogram increase. Total-body strength increases were greater when 3.0 grams of HMB were used (Figure 10-1). In addition, less protein degradation and muscle damage was observed in the group consuming 3.0 grams of HMB.

Since that study was conducted in 1996, approximately half of subsequent studies have shown HMB to be ergogenic (Figure 10-2). Interestingly, many of the studies showing ergogenicity used lesser-trained individuals, while several studies showing no ergogenic effects were completed using strength-trained athletes. A meta-analysis of HMB studies (Nissen and Sharp, 2003) showed supplementation with 3.0 grams of HMB per day was ergogenic and resulted in approximately a 1.4 percent strength increase per week. In addition to performance enhancement, some studies have shown HMB actually reduced muscle damage during running and strength training,

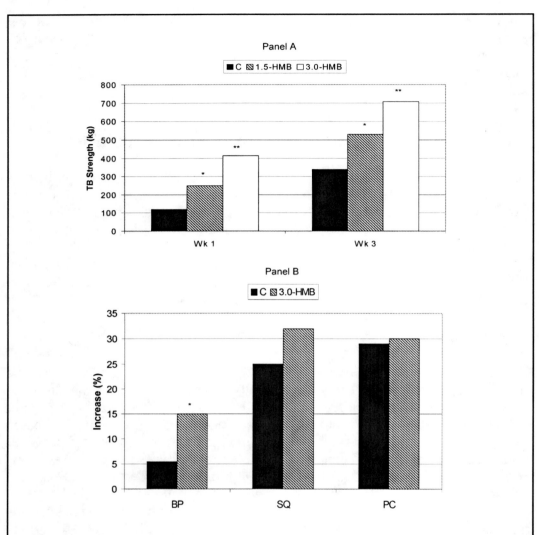

Panel A: This graph shows the changes after one and three weeks of supplementation with either 1.5 or 3.0 grams of HMB per day. Dose-dependent strength gains were seen in the total amount of weight lifted for the total body (TB).

Panel B: This graph shows the percent changes in 1 RM bench press (BP), squat (SQ), and power clean (PC) following 7 weeks of training with a placebo or 3.0 grams of HMB per day. Although slightly greater increases were seen in all three exercises, only the changes seen in the bench press were significant.

* = greater than control; ** = greater than control and 1.5 grams of HMB per day

Figures modified from Nissen and colleagues (1996).

Figure 10-1. Strength changes with HMB supplementation

while one study did not show any reductions in muscle damage following an intense eccentric-exercise protocol. Clearly, not all studies have shown HMB to be ergogenic. However, strength and power athletes who are attempting to increase size and strength may consider supplementation with HMB with at least 3 to 6 grams per day in divided doses (three to four per day). Several multipurpose supplements include HMB. For example, Jowko and colleagues (2001) found an additive effect of creatine-plus-HMB that was better than that of either creatine or HMB alone. HMB supplementation is legal and no adverse side effects have been reported. In fact, HMB supplementation has been shown to reduce total cholesterol, LDL cholesterol, and systolic blood pressure.

Reference	Subjects	Sup. Regimen	Results
Kreider et al., 1999	RT athletes	3 or 6 grams of HMB/day for 28 days plus RT	↔ 1 RM BP, LP ***Not ergogenic**
Panton et al., 2000	UT & T men and women	3.0 grams of HMB/day for 4 weeks plus RT	↑ UB strength and LBM, ↓ percent fat *****Ergogenic**
Gallagher et al., 2000	UT men	0, 3, or 6 grams of HMB/day for 8 weeks plus RT	3 grams: ↑ ISOM torque, LBM > 0 or 6 grams 6 grams: ↑ ISOK torque > 0 or 3 grams ↔ 1 RM, % fat *****Ergogenic**
Slater et al., 2001	RT M athletes	3 grams of HMB/day for 6 weeks plus RT	↔ 3 RM strength, LBM ***Not ergogenic**
Vukovich et al., 2001	UT elderly M, F	3 grams of HMB/day for 8 weeks plus RT	↑ LBM, ↓ percent fat *****Ergogenic**
Ransone et al., 2003	College FB players	3 grams of HMB/day for 4 weeks plus RT	↔ BP, SQ, PC strength, LBM, percent fat ***Not ergogenic**
Hoffman et al., 2004	College FB players	3 grams of HMB/day for 10 days during FB camp	↔ anaerobic power ***Not ergogenic**
Thomson, 2004	RT men	3 grams of HMB/day for 9 weeks plus RT	↑ LE strength; ↔ body composition *****Ergogenic**

Note: ↑ = HMB resulted in greater increases; ↔ = HBM provided no further benefit; ↓ = HMB resulted in a greater reduction; RT = resistance training; UT = untrained; T = trained; FB = football; M = male; F = female; BP = bench press; LP = leg press; UB = upper body; LBM = lean body mass; ISOM = isometric; ISOK = isokinetic; PC = power clean; SQ = squat; LE = leg extension

Figure 10-2. HMB supplementation and performance

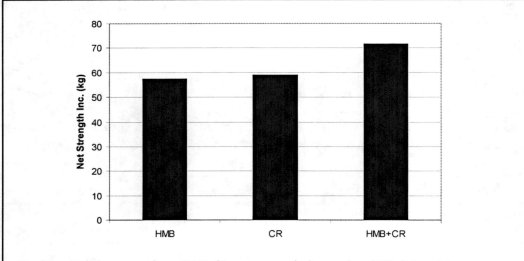

Total strength increases from HMB (3 grams per day), creatine (CR) (10 to 20 grams per day), and HMB-plus-CR for 3 weeks.

Figure modified from Jowko et al. (2001).

Figure 10-3. Strength increases with HMB, creatine, and HMB-plus-creatine

ß-Alanine and Carnosine

Carnosine, a dipeptide consisting of β-alanine and L-histidine, is a major skeletal-muscle buffer, meaning that it neutralizes elevated H^+ during exercise. It is found in both fast-twitch and slow-twitch muscle fibers, though in twice the concentration in fast-twitch fibers. Suzuki and colleagues (2002) have shown that individuals with high muscle carnosine content perform better during the latter half of a 30-second maximal cycle sprint. Very little research has examined carnosine supplementation on anaerobic performance. One study (Kraemer et al., 1995) looked at Phosfuel™, which contains predominantly inorganic phosphates, bicarbonate, and carnosine and found that it did not improve repetitive maximal cycling performance. However, it did improve peak power recovery.

Increasing the concentrations of β-alanine can lead to greater synthesis of carnosine. In horses, oral L-histidine and β-alanine increased muscle carnosine content. β-alanine supplements are increasing in popularity, but little research has been performed. We conducted a study at The College of New Jersey examining a combined β-alanine and creatine supplement and found that the combination resulted in a greater resistance-training response (i.e., loads lifted, training volume) than creatine supplementation alone. Although some promise appears to be evident with combined creatine and β-alanine supplementation, more research is needed before any recommendations can be made.

Citrulline Malate

This combination supplement consists of *citrulline*, which is involved in urea metabolism and accelerates the rate of urea and lactate metabolism, and *malate*, which is an aerobic-system intermediate. It is thought that this supplement can reduce fatigue, reduce lactate concentrations, perhaps increase nitric oxide levels, and increase energy contribution from aerobic metabolism. In Europe, this supplement has been used to treat fatigue and muscle weakness. Some evidence shows citrulline malate supplementation (6 grams per day for 15 days) increases the aerobic-energy system's contribution to exercise and enhanced recovery, although some methodological concerns make it difficult to state if a definitive ergogenic potential to citrulline malate exists. Citrulline and malate are found in high concentrations in melons and apples, respectively. Many athletes have supplemented with 3 to 6 grams per day, but more research is certainly necessary before recommendations can be made.

Cortitrol™

Cortitrol is a supplement consisting of several vitamins and minerals and a proprietary herbal blend of anticortisol agents, including magnolia bark extract (*magnolia officialis*, which suppresses cortisol), L-theanine (from *camillia sinensis*, an immune-system enhancer), epimedium extract (*epimedium koreanum*, which suppresses cortisol), phophatidylserine (a cortisol suppressant), and beta-sitosterol (improves prostate health and lowers cholesterol). While the hormone cortisol is necessary to respond to physiological stress, chronic elevation of cortisol may have negative effects such as reduced immune-cell function, greater protein breakdown in muscle, and reduced bone metabolism. These effects may be particularly evident in an athlete who encounters a great deal of stress from training, practice, competition, school, etc. At the University of Connecticut, we examined Cortitrol supplementation in strength-trained men following a highly stressful protocol (i.e., four sets of 10 repetitions of four multiple-joint exercises with two-minute rest intervals) and found cortisol and free-radical concentrations were reduced with Cortitrol supplementation. These initial results show some promise for Cortitrol supplementation in athletes, but further research is needed.

Glucosamine-Chondroitin and Hyaluronic Acid

Glucosamine and chondroitin sulfate are substances found naturally in the human body. Glucosamine is a form of amino sugar that plays a role in cartilage formation and

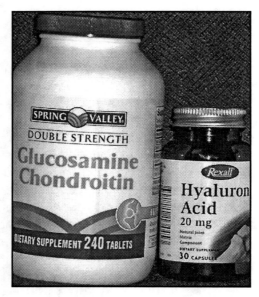

Figure 10-4. Glucosamine-chondroitin and hyaluronic-acid supplements

repair. Chondroitin sulfate is a proteoglycan that gives cartilage its elasticity and prevents other body enzymes from degrading joint cartilage. Both are extracted from animal tissue—glucosamine from crab, lobster, or shrimp shells and chondroitin sulfate from animal cartilage, such as tracheas or shark cartilage. Another key connective-tissue component of synovial, or joint, fluid that acts as a joint lubricant is *hyaluronic acid*, which has been used in supplemental form to treat and/or prevent joint deterioration. Although hyaluronic-acid injections have shown some promise in treating osteoarthritis, oral supplementation remains limited in its effects. Some studies have shown that glucosamine-chondroitin supplementation can reduce cartilage degeneration and help improve symptoms of osteoarthritis in the knees, hips, and intervertebral disks. Although some studies refute this finding, it appears that some potential may exist to help joint integrity in athletes.

Many supplements include glucosamine (approximately 1,500 milligrams) and chondroitin sulfate (approximately 1,200 milligrams). Glucosamine-chondroitin sulfate may not be ergogenic per se. However, the potential to reduce future problems may be attractive from a supplementation standpoint. For example, studies have shown that athletes are at a greater risk for osteoarthritis later in life when compared to nonathletes. In fact, the incidence of hip, knee, and ankle osteoarthritis is higher in athletes, especially those involved in power or mixed-power sports that require sporadic power bursts. Therefore, glucosamine-chondroitin supplementation may be viewed as "preventative" rather than ergogenic.

Glutamine

Glutamine is a nonessential amino acid that is readily synthesized in several tissues within the body from glutamate, which itself is synthesized from alpha-ketoglutarate. It has several roles that make supplementation attractive. Glutamine is an important fuel for immune cells. Glutamine produced in the muscles passes through the muscle membrane into the blood to maintain adequate glutamine levels. This action is critical because low blood glutamine levels are linked to compromised immune function. Short-duration, moderate-to-high intensity exercise (e.g., sprints) may result in higher blood glutamine levels, whereas exhaustive, long-duration exercise (e.g., marathons) results in much lower blood glutamine levels. Therefore, strenuous exercise resulting in great metabolic stress and muscle damage compromises immune function and places the athlete at a greater risk for infection. In fact, a higher incidence of upper respiratory tract infections in endurance athletes has been shown.

Glutamine supplementation can increase blood levels of glutamine and improve immune-system function. It has been shown that taking 0.1 grams per kilogram of body mass of glutamine for seven days resulted in a 32-percent reduction in the likelihood of suffering an upper respiratory tract infection following a marathon. Since athletes need to compete and train very intensely (and subsequently run the risk of overtraining, which also limits immune-system function), glutamine supplementation may be advantageous during stressful training to reduce the risk of illness.

Glutamine is also important for maintaining skeletal muscle protein content (possibly increasing synthesis and reducing breakdown), increasing glucose metabolism, and facilitating the synthesis of glucosamine. It is thought that glutamine can increase muscle protein synthesis—possibly through a mechanism similar to that of creatine—by increasing water content (making it a "cell volumizer"). An increase in water content leads to a series of events that increase protein synthesis. On the other hand, studies have also found a limited ergogenicity of glutamine supplementation in athletes. Six weeks of combined strength training and glutamine supplementation (0.9 grams per kilogram of lean body mass) did not result in any greater gains in muscle strength or lean-tissue mass. The combination of creatine and glutamine has been shown to be ergogenic for increasing power and lean-body mass. However, the improvements were similar to supplementing with creatine alone, thereby showing the limited effects of the addition of glutamine. Although supplementation with glutamine has physiological relevance, research hasn't shown enhanced performance. Because of glutamine's immune system–enhancing function during stressful training, athletes may benefit from supplementation. Many multipurpose supplements on the market contain glutamine in great abundance. Glutamine supplementation has been shown to be safe in the short-term, typically with supplementation of 5 to 20 grams per day.

Ornithine Alpha Ketoglutarate

Ornithine alpha-ketoglutarate (OKG) is a salt formed from alpha-ketoglutarate and two molecules of ornithine. This combination, which is used to treat trauma such as burn injuries, may have a synergistic role in reducing muscle-protein breakdown and increasing protein synthesis, possibly due to increased secretion of insulin and human growth hormone or the synthesis (or sparing) of glutamine, arginine, and proline. OKG has a more potent effect on glutamine synthesis than A-AKG. Similar to glutamine, it is thought that OKG supplementation may be most effective during stressful situations for athletes (e.g., when overtraining, during injury).

Chetlin and colleagues (2000) conducted a study with healthy, strength-trained men. They investigated the effects of 10 grams of OKG (with 75 grams of CHO) and showed that it did not alter growth-hormone and insulin response. After six weeks of strength training, similar results were obtained when examining workout performance and one-repetition maximum (1 RM) squat performance. However, OKG supplementation (10 grams per day) enhanced 1 RM bench press to a greater extent. It is difficult to explain these findings and to determine if, in fact, OKG can be ergogenic for athletic performance. It appears most effective in times of high stress, and may play less of a role during normal training in healthy athletes. OKG supplementation appears safe at approximately 10 grams per day, but higher doses could cause some mild gastric distress.

Octacosanol

Octacosanol is a 28-carbon long-chain waxy alcohol found in wheat germ oil. It appears to play a role in lowering LDL cholesterol levels by more than 25 percent and raising HDL levels by up to 15 percent, and may have some antioxidant functions due to its high vitamin E content. In rats, octacosanol supplementation increased running endurance by 46 percent by enhancing oxidative capacity and sparing muscle glycogen stores. In humans, 1 milligram per day given over eight weeks resulted in greater reaction time and grip strength, but not chest strength or cycling endurance. More research is needed to evaluate this supplement. Octacosanol supplements typically contain 8 to 20 milligrams to be taken per day. No adverse effects are yet known, but its use as an ergogenic supplement is questionable despite some health-promoting benefits.

Pyruvate

Pyruvate is a three-carbon compound formed during the metabolism of carbohydrates that has two possible fates. It is either converted to lactic acid during high-intensity exercise or acts as a precursor to acetyl-CoA, which is critical to aerobic energy metabolism. In some studies, the combination of pyruvate and dihydroxyacetone (another metabolic intermediate) supplementation has yielded some positive, yet controversial, results. Pyruvate (and dihydroxyacetone) has been shown to increase fat breakdown, reduce fat storage, and lower levels of insulin. In addition, pyruvate-supplemented animals and humans (typically with 6 to 44 grams per day for six weeks) have lost more body fat and weight than with a placebo.

Pyruvate's potential to enhance performance is critical to athletes. Large doses (100 grams of pyruvate and dihydroxyacetone plus high carbohydrate intake) consumed over seven days has been shown to increase muscle glycogen by 48 percent and increase arm and leg cycle-ergometer endurance by 20 to 23 percent, respectively, in untrained subjects. However, lower doses (i.e., 7 to 25 grams) of calcium pyruvate (which is still somewhat more than typically recommended by supplement manufacturers) in trained male cyclists did not enhance cycling performance, nor did it substantially increase blood pyruvate levels. Those lower doses also did not enhance exercise performance or reduce body fat in untrained women.

Creatine and combined creatine-plus-pyruvate supplementation (9 grams per day) has been shown to enhance body composition, strength, and power in football players. However, the addition of pyruvate to creatine does not produce any ergogenic effects. Therefore, it may be possible that pyruvate is ergogenic at higher doses, but may not be worth consuming due to the amount of potential stomach distress. These ergogenic studies did not examine pyruvate alone, which is typically how it is sold in supplement stores (i.e., commercial supplements do not typically contain dihydroxyacetone and instead contain approximately 3 to 6 grams of pyruvate only). Therefore, the verdict is still out on pyruvate and many experts do not recommend its use.

Ribose

Ribose is a sugar that is formed from the conversion of glucose via the pentose phosphate pathway. During energy production from adenosine triphosphate (ATP) breakdown, adenosine diphosphate (ADP) is formed in high quantities, of which a fraction is subsequently degraded to inosine 5'-monophosphate (IMP), inosine, and hypoxanthine. The rate of breakdown is related to the intensity and duration of exercise, so that ATP is depleted quickly. The key to recovery is the reversal of this process. Making the process of recovery more difficult, some inosine and hypoxanthine can exit muscle and enter the blood, meaning that these lost compounds need to be restored. Recovery is typically slow. Therefore, finding a way to increase the rate of recovery is important for any athlete.

Increasing the rate at which hypoxanthine converts to IMP ultimately results in the resynthesis of the body's main energy compound, ATP. In addition, increasing de novo synthesis (newly synthesized compound from precursors) restores these nucleotides and gives athletes more energy to train and compete. The formation of ribose-5-phosphate increases the rate at which IMP, and subsequently ATP, is synthesized. It is thought that this step may be a limiting factor during high-intensity exercise. Ribose supplementation is thought to push these reactions in the reverse direction and ultimately increase the rate of ATP resynthesis as well as the athlete's ability to sustain high-intensity exercise. This effect is critical because high-intensity exercise performed over several days can reduce muscle ATP levels by 20 to 25 percent, and this depletion may not completely recover until three days later. Ribose is rapidly absorbed from the intestines and is well-tolerated at high doses, which make it easily consumed prior to, or during, an exercise bout.

For a ribose supplement to work, it needs to be readily transported into skeletal muscle. Although it appears that ribose can get to its target destination relatively quickly, its potential for ergogenicity has yielded conflicting results. Ribose supplementation of 16 grams per day over six days has not been found to reduce fatigue or enhance power and force performance of repeated maximal knee extensions. It also did not increase ATP recovery. Interestingly, consumption of 200 milligrams per kilogram of body mass of ribose for three days was shown to increase the rate of ATP recovery by 72 hours postexercise, but did not enhance performance of 15 10-second cycle sprints. In contrast, some evidence of greater work performance and reduced fatigue has been shown with 10 to 32 grams per day of ribose during intermittent cycle sprints, although many other performance variables were not enhanced.

In another study (Antonio and Stout, 2002), bodybuilders were given either a placebo or 5 grams of ribose 15 minutes before a workout and 5 grams five minutes after the workout. The ribose group improved bench-press performance by approximately 20 percent, while the placebo group improved by 12 percent. Therefore, some evidence does indicate that ribose supplementation may help maintain performance during high-intensity exercise. Although some studies do not support these findings, athletes may consider giving ribose a try prior to training or competition. Some athletes respond well, while others will see no benefits. A particular athlete's response may not be known until he experiments with ribose at the recommended doses. It is recommended that ribose supplementation (10 to 15 grams per day) be split into smaller doses (5 grams each) and taken with a carbohydrate beverage before, during, or immediately after a strenuous workout. Ribose supplementation is legal and does not appear to yield any negative side effects at the recommended doses.

Coaching Points

- *Definitely worth a try*: Nitric oxide boosters, β-HMB, glucosamine-chondroitin, glutamine, ribose
- *Some possible potential*: L-carnitine, β-alanine, Cortitrol, citrulline malate, OKG
- *May not be worth it*: Octacosanol, pyruvate

11

Anabolic Agents

Athletes commonly use anabolic agents to enhance performance. While these "agents" are classified as drugs and require a prescription, unfortunately they are illegally used and abused by many athletes. Historically, strength and power athletes (e.g., track and field athletes, weightlifters, bodybuilders, power lifters, and football players) were the predominant users of these drugs. However, with the many advances in the strength and conditioning profession, use of these drugs spread, and athletes from most sports have been known to experiment with them. The anabolic agents discussed in this chapter are anabolic steroids and testosterone derivatives, human growth hormone, insulin, insulin-like growth factor-1, human chorionic gonadotropin (HCG), and clenbuterol.

Anabolic Steroids

What Are Anabolic Steroids?

Anabolic steroids are synthetic derivatives of the hormone testosterone, which, in addition to its anabolic (i.e., tissue-building) properties, possesses androgenic properties. For this reason, some experts in the field refer to them as *anabolic-androgenic steroids*. The androgenic effects relate to testosterone's role in the development of secondary sexual characteristics and the reproductive system. Athletes use anabolic steroids for their ergogenic properties (Figure 11-1). However, many athletes attempt to reduce the androgenic effects using several methods, including using low-androgenic steroids, injectable steroids, or other drugs.

Although training alone results in acute elevations in testosterone, the magnitude is far less than what might be attained with drug (i.e., anabolic steroid or testosterone)

- Increased lean-body mass
- Increased cardiac-tissue mass
- Decreased body-fat percent
- Increased isometric and dynamic muscle strength and power
- Enhanced recovery ability between workouts and from injuries
- Increased protein synthesis
- Increased muscle cross-sectional area
- Stimulated growth of the epiphysial plate
- Increased erythropoiesis, hemoglobin, and hematocrit
- Increased bone-mineral density
- Increased glycogen storage
- Increased lipolysis
- Increased neural transmission
- Increased pain tolerance
- Behaviour modification (i.e., aggression)

Figure 11-1. General effects of anabolic steroids

use. In addition, natural testosterone (produced by the Leydig cells of the testes under the regulation of a hormone called *luteinizing hormone*) has a short half-life in the human body and is broken down rapidly by the liver. Therefore, biochemical modification of testosterone can increase its half-life and its potency. Several different biochemical alterations may be made and a wide variety of anabolic steroids are used by athletes. The overall net effects depend on the structure of the steroid, how long it remains active, and how it interacts with the *androgen receptor*, which is the protein receptor in tissues that regulates the functions of testosterone. Anabolic steroids with long half-lives and moderate-to-strong interactions with the androgen receptor possess greater potential for anabolic and androgenic effects at lower administration doses. It is important that you do not confuse anabolic steroids with the anti-inflammatory steroids that are commonly prescribed for injuries. These steroids reduce inflammation and have no anabolic/androgenic properties.

Incidence of Anabolic Steroid Use

Despite being classified as a Schedule III Controlled Substance and illegal to purchase without medicinal purposes (i.e., a prescription) and banned from most sport governing bodies, the use of anabolic steroids in athletes has increased over the years. It has been estimated that more than three million anabolic steroid users exist in the United States, many of whom are competitive athletes or recreational bodybuilders. Since testosterone was isolated chemically in 1935, interest in this hormone for enhancing performance (and aggression) has steadily increased. Historically, anabolic steroid use began in the mid-1950s in the United States (although some experimentation may have taken place earlier). The weightlifting community popularized anabolic steroid use, but it spread to other sports such as track and field and football in the early 1960s. Unfortunately, modern athletes of all ages and in most sports have experimented with anabolic steroids.

Several self-report and survey studies have provided estimates of anabolic steroid use among athletes of different sports. It is important to note that some estimates may be drastically lower than the actual amount because of the unwillingness of athletes to admit steroid use and other methodological issues associated with surveys. Interestingly, when athletes are surveyed to estimate steroid use among their competitors, the numbers are significantly higher than what is reported by the athletes themselves. In addition, drug testing has failed to provide insight into the incidence of steroid use because very few athletes have tested positive (the limitations of drug testing are discussed later in this chapter). Yesalis and colleagues (2000) reviewed the literature and categorized many of these studies. Reports have shown that, of the responders, 0.7 to 6.3 percent of male adolescents and 0.1 to 3.2 percent of female adolescents have reported some type of anabolic steroid use. Several studies have examined anabolic steroid use in college athletes. These studies (dating back to 1985) have reported the following incidence of use among athletes of different sports (approximately 25,000 sampled):

Football—2.2 to 9.7 percent

Men's track and field—0 to 4.7 percent

Men's basketball—0.6 to 3.6 percent

Men's tennis—0 to 3.6 percent

Softball—0 to 1.7 percent

Baseball—0.7 to 3.5 percent

Women's track and field—0 to 2.7 percent

Women's basketball—0 to 1.5 percent

Women's tennis—0 to 2.7 percent

Women's swimming—0.6 to 1 percent

The higher the level of competition, the higher the incidence of anabolic steroid use. Reports from elite-level weightlifters, bodybuilders, power lifters, and track and field athletes have shown an incidence of use ranging from 31 to 68 percent. In fact, Taylor (2002) estimated the incidence of steroid use to be 95 to 100 percent among professional body builders, wrestlers, and heavyweight boxers; 65 to 70 percent among professional football players; and 20 to 25 percent among professional basketball and baseball players. In addition, personal accounts from athletes participating in different sports have estimated anabolic steroid use to be much higher than those reported in previous studies. In fact, the general consensus among elite strength and power athletes is that it would be far more difficult to find an athlete who has never used steroids than identify those who have. Clearly, anabolic steroid use is rampant in sports and very little is being done to handle the problem.

As stated previously, many athletes have illegally experimented with anabolic steroids. The key term here is "experimented," as most information used to quantify steroid use is anecdotal and based on the testimony of other users or teammates. For ethical reasons, science has virtually ignored the use of steroids with the intent of improving athletic performance, instead focusing on clinical uses. Thus, athletes committed to using anabolic steroids sought information from anyone who had some knowledge or experience. Unfortunately, the quest to experimentally find optimal "anabolic drug stacks and cycles" has replaced the quest to maximize training-program design in some circles. Nevertheless, once resistance training gained acceptance among athletes, anabolic steroid use was not far behind, owing to the benefits of enhanced muscular strength, power, mass, and endurance.

Types of Anabolic Steroids and Methods of Use

Anabolic steroids are testosterone derivatives. Testosterone consists of four rings with several numbered carbons. The potency of testosterone and testosterone derivatives depends upon several factors, including its half life, interaction with the *androgen receptor*, and the interaction with binding proteins. In addition, a key element to the potency of anabolic steroids is the capacity for synergistic effects with other drugs consumed (e.g., growth hormone, insulin). Therefore, some testosterone derivatives have been biochemically altered (mainly at the α and β positions of the 17th carbon, and the 2nd, 9th, 11th, and 19th carbon positions) to remain in the system longer and interact with the receptor to a greater magnitude. These derivatives tend to produce more substantial effects, which can be *anabolic* when the target tissues are skeletal muscle or bone, but also may be *androgenic* when other tissues are affected.

The anabolic effects are desired. However, athletes attempt to minimize the androgenic effects (see the "Side Effects" section in this chapter) via steroid selection or by taking other drugs (antiestrogens). No single anabolic steroid exists that is purely anabolic with no androgenic effects. In some cases, a *therapeutic index* may be used to describe the ratio of anabolic to androgenic effects. For example, a steroid such as nandrolone decanoate (Deca Durabolin) has an index of 11:1 to 12:1 and possesses a ratio favoring anabolism to a far greater extent than testosterone cypionate (Depo-Testosterone), which has a ratio of 1:1, meaning it has equal anabolic and androgenic properties.

Anabolic steroids come in different forms. *Oral anabolic steroids* are taken by mouth and tend to have half-lives (i.e., the time blood values return to half of the original concentration within the athlete) of a few to several hours, which is shorter than injectable steroids. Oral steroids, therefore, are taken more frequently (one or more

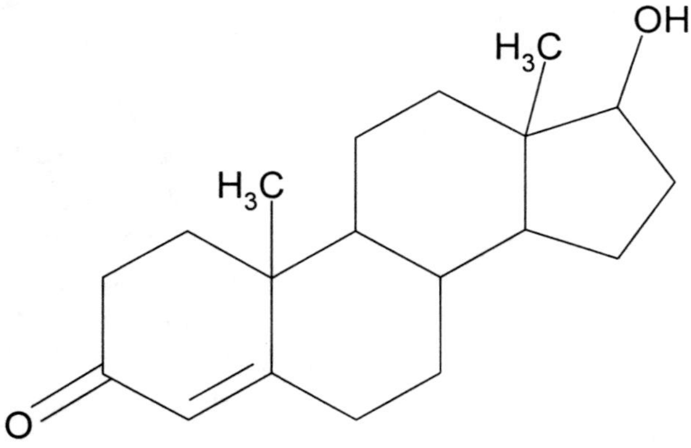

Alterations of this basic structure can increase the potency and half-life of testosterone, thereby chemically paving the way for numerous anabolic drugs commonly used by athletes.

Figure 11-2. Chemical structure of testosterone

times daily) and are more toxic to the liver. Oral steroids are mostly 17-alpha alkylated variations, which increase protection against stomach acids during digestion and degradation by the liver during "first pass," as they must first be absorbed through the gastrointestinal tract. Some commonly used and abused oral steroids are Anavar, Winstrol, Dianabol, and Halotestin.

Injectable steroids come in two forms, oil-based and water-based. *Oil-based injectable* steroids are modified at the 17-beta position to make them more soluble in lipids and oils. The longer the side chain, the longer the steroid remains in the athlete's body. These steroids are injected deep into skeletal muscle (in an oil vehicle) and have much longer half-lives than oral forms (i.e., several days to a week). Consequently, an athlete may use oil-based injectable steroids on a weekly basis. Some examples are Deca Durabolin and Depo-Testosterone. In addition, some oil-based injectable steroids are modified at the 19th carbon, which tends to promote anabolism (e.g., Deca Durabolin).

Water-based injectable steroids have half-lives similar to oral forms (i.e., several hours) and may be injected several times weekly. These steroids typically cause less discomfort and many times are used to reduce body fat in addition to anabolism. Some examples are Winstrol-V and testosterone suspension. Other preparations include testosterone patches and gels, buccal tablets, nasal sprays, and creams. In many cases, athletes have reported beginning use with oral steroids, but progressing to injectables once their comfort levels increase regarding drug use. A survey examining drug-use patterns among 500 anabolic steroid users showed that 99.2 percent of the participants used either injectable or a combination of oral and injectable steroids (Parkinson and Evans, 2006).

Another prime concern for the athlete is the amount of time anabolic steroids can be detected in the human body. Oral steroids and some water-based injectables typically remain in the body for a short-to-moderate time. For example, testosterone suspension may stay in the system for one to three days, while other testosterone preparations (e.g., testosterone propionate and undeconoate) may stay in the system for a few weeks. Some orals such as Dianabol, Anavar, and Winstrol (tablets) may stay in the system for three to six weeks. Other steroids such as Halotestin, Anadrol-50, Sustanon-250, Winstrol-V, Testosterone Cypionate, and Enanthate may stay in the system for two to three months. Oil-based steroids such as Deca Durabolin and Durabolin may stay in the system for 12 to 18 months. The exact amount of time depends on the volume and frequency of use, as well as the athlete's history and pattern of prior use. An athlete could fail a drug test within these time periods if anabolic steroids are used, which could be a major deterrent for use.

Athletes use anabolic steroids in various ways. Typically, an athlete will initially experiment with one anabolic steroid. He then may move on to *cycle* steroids to maximize the effects and minimize some side effects. Many such cycles are five to 12 weeks in duration (and longer in some cases). Parkinson and Evans (2006) reported that 93 percent of steroid users sampled used a cyclical pattern of use, while 6 percent consumed consistent doses over a one-year period. Long-term steroid use could result in a large downregulation of the androgen receptors, thereby leading to a higher *tolerance*. When this happens, larger doses are needed to elicit a similar effect. At this point, the athlete increases the dose, which ultimately turns into steroid abuse as he exceeds the typical dose-response relationship.

When anabolic steroids are cycled, a pattern of increasing use on a weekly basis usually occurs, although some athletes consume a steady dose but cycle the drugs being consumed. This pattern is usually followed by a one- to two-week period of maintenance at that dose and then a few weeks of gradual reduction until use of the drug is ceased for some period of time. During the down-cycle, androgen-receptor function is restored and the body's natural ability to synthesize and secrete testosterone is brought back to homeostatic levels. Although some athletes may take a constant dose for several weeks or even sporadically use anabolic steroids, cycling is the preferred method for most athletes. Many athletes will take multiple anabolic steroids or other drugs in a process known as stacking. With stacking, more than one steroid is taken in a cyclical fashion to amplify the effects. In fact, Perry et al. (2005) showed that the athletes surveyed averaged 3.1 drugs in a stack and Parkinson and Evans (2006) showed that 95 percent of steroid users sampled used at least two different anabolic steroids.

Anabolic steroids, as well as other anabolic agents, work in synergy when taken together. In other words, use of one type may amplify the effects of another. To minimize the potential lost effects resulting from reduced steroid use, some athletes will *stagger* steroids so that they down-cycle on one type but initiate another cycle for a different steroid. Although many athletes are "scientific" when designing their anabolic steroid cycles, others take many forms at high doses in a hit-or-miss manner (called the shotgun method). It is important to note that science has not effectively addressed these various methods of steroid use for athletic purposes. Therefore, the information athletes are using typically comes from reading magazines, websites, books, or advice/testimonials from friends, teammates, or other athletes or gym members.

In the "gym world," information is shared on the efficacy of various forms of steroids. Again, science has not really examined this information, as much of it is anecdotal and based on the successes and failures of other athletes who have experimented themselves or received information from other steroid users. For example, steroids such as Anadrol, Anavar, Dianabol, Sustanon-250, various testosterone preparations, and Deca Durabolin are thought of as effective in increasing muscle mass and strength. Other steroids such as Winstrol-V, Parabolan, and Primobolan Depot are thought to have "cutting" effects. A large part of training in athletes who use anabolic steroids focuses on seeking more beneficial cycles of properly stacked agents to increase performance. In addition, the doses athletes have used far exceed clinical recommendations by five to 100 times, which poses major health concerns to individuals consuming anabolic steroids.

Designer Steroids

Chemists have altered testosterone to develop new derivatives—*designer steroids*—that have anabolic potential, but cannot be detected through testing unless they are specifically sought. These steroids are not on the market and are not tested for. The incident involving designer steroids that has received the most attention is the BALCO case, in which several professional athletes were supplied with a designer steroid, tetrahydrogestrinone (THG), and a testosterone cream to avoid any possibility of detection. Other steroids, such as norbolethone and Madol, which were not known to be on the market, have turned up in the urine of some athletes as well. As designer steroids become well-known, they will ultimately be added to the list of banned substances. However, athletes (and chemists) typically are ahead of the game. As authorities develop more stringent testing for these designer steroids, other designer steroids will undoubtedly replace them.

Sources of Steroids

Athletes obtain anabolic steroids from several sources. Without a prescription for medicinal purposes, anabolic steroids are illegal and banned from athletic competition.

However, athletes may obtain steroids from dealers at local gyms or other athletes (i.e., on the black market). The sales or distribution of anabolic steroids in this fashion is a crime. Results of a survey of 500 anabolic steroid users showed that 89 percent of steroids were obtained illegally (e.g., from gym members/dealers, Internet dealers, mail order, and bootleg laboratories), whereas 11 percent were obtained via prescription from a physician.

Steroids obtained on the black market typically are lower in cost. However, an athlete cannot be 100 percent certain about what he is purchasing. Counterfeit steroids are commonly sold on the black market. They look similar to real steroids, but have no beneficial effects. Some athletes may even venture to Mexico, where anabolic steroids can be legally purchased over the counter. In some cases, physicians or medical professionals will prescribe or personally provide anabolic steroids to athletes for nonmedicinal purposes. The government has cracked down on this practice and a physician can face steep punishment if found guilty. The purchase of anabolic steroids from a pharmacy is certainly legal if a person has a prescription. However, most physicians will not take the risk of providing athletes with opportunities to purchase anabolic steroids.

Steroids have also been sold through the mail. This practice was made easier through the advent of the Internet. Anabolic steroids can be ordered on some websites, especially from pharmacies in other countries. Some websites will even supply a prescription to "legalize" the transaction. Regardless of the method of purchase, anabolic steroid use is prohibited and athletes can face steep penalties if caught.

Ergogenic Effects

As shown in Figure 11-1, anabolic steroids have many ergogenic effects that can enhance athletic performance. In the athletic community, it is well-accepted that anabolic steroids work very well. However, the results of some research studies leave some scientists unconvinced that steroids are ergogenic. In fact, between 1977 and 1984, the American College of Sports Medicine regarded steroids as ineffective. Several studies have since been published showing the large ergogenic potential of these drugs. It is important to note that carefully controlled scientific studies typically elucidate the effects of one anabolic steroid at clinical doses. However, athletes' use of anabolic steroids differs substantially from this protocol. Therefore, it is not surprising than that the gains in performance reported by anabolic steroid users far exceed those reported in the scientific literature. Some factors that may contribute to the potentiated ergogenic effects (as compared to those found in research studies) are as follows:

- Athletes reportedly consume anabolic steroids in doses far greater than those clinically recommended or those examined in many studies.

- Athletes stack different anabolic steroids (and other anabolic agents and supplements), which may have a synergistic effect and compound the ergogenic effects. Note that research studies generally examine the isolated effects of one steroid.

- Athletes consume additional kilocalories, including greater carbohydrate and protein intake, when cycling steroids, which can increase the anabolic response. Note that scientists control diets and monitor kilocalorie intake during research studies.

- Athletes train at a higher level during steroid use, which could lead to greater ergogenic effects. The training intensity/volume used in clinical studies does not match the type/amount of training followed by athletes.

Side Effects

Anabolic steroids have numerous side effects (Figure 11-3), some of which appear to be more prevalent with oral steroid use. However, long-term use of either oral or injectable anabolic steroids can be problematic. Anabolic steroids taken at clinically recommended doses under physician supervision appear to be safe. However, when steroids are taken beyond these recommendations for long periods, side effects may persist. Although many of these effects are reversible upon discontinuance of steroid use, some long-term damage could occur. In addition, many anabolic steroid users (approximately 96 percent) consume other prescription drugs, including those meant to reduce potential side effects from the steroids themselves, rather than discontinue steroid use. Therefore, some experts fear anabolic steroid use may serve as a "gateway" to other drug use, including recreational use. It appears that side effects are imminent, as approximately 99 percent of anabolic steroid users have reported at least one side effect, while approximately 70 percent have reported at least three side effects. Lastly, injectable-steroid users have reported hazardous injection procedures, such as reusing needles (13 percent), sharing vials (8 percent), and sharing needles with others (1 percent), which increase the risk of disease. Most anabolic steroid users are aware of the potential dangers and are concerned about side effects (more than 60 percent). However, these dangers do not appear to supersede the quest for ergogenicity, as it appears larger risks are being taken in comparison to steroid use during previous decades.

Steroid Testing

Steroid testing has been instituted in an attempt to create a "fair and level playing field." However, it has been a failure in most cases. Many sport-governing bodies implement steroid testing for political reasons—to demonstrate to the public that it is concerned about fair play, enforcing the law, and protecting the health of the athletes. In reality, this reasoning is mostly rhetoric, as a severe lack of commitment (and often funding) exists to rid sports of anabolic steroids. Steroid testing can almost be viewed as a "no win"

Male

Reduction in testicular size/function
Reduced sperm count
Lower levels of natural testosterone
Gynecomastia
Benign prostate enlargement

Female

Clitoral enlargement
Reduction in breast tissue
Menstrual disturbances
Masculinization

Both Genders

Male-pattern baldness	Hypertension
Acne	Deepening of voice
Fluid retention	Abnormal liver function
Increased libido	Increased body and facial hair
Altered thyroid function	Nose bleeds
Aggression	Psychological disturbance
Greater appetite	Insulin resistance
Glucose intolerance	Peliosis hepatitis
Increased sebaceous gland secretions	Blood clotting abnormalities
Increased LDL	Decreased HDL
Higher total cholesterol	Liver damage/disease
Greater risk for heart attack and stroke	Atherosclerosis
Skin rash	Heart hypertrophy
Premature growth plate closure (adolescents)	Avascular necrosis
Greater risk for tendon/ligament injuries	Headaches
Depression	Dizziness
Mood swings	Greater risk for cancer
Violent tendencies ("roid rage")	Kidney abnormalities
Drug dependence	Higher estrogen levels
Other infections/disease from needle sharing	

Figure 11-3. Side effects associated with anabolic steroid use

situation for the governing bodies. On one hand, if many athletes fail the drug tests (and the results are not covered up as part of a scandal), the testing procedures look promising, but a true drug problem has been exposed, giving the sport a very poor image. On the other hand, if few athletes fail drug tests, it appears that the testing procedures are limited, especially when reports from athletes offer strategies for beating the tests while anecdotally estimating large numbers of athletes using these drugs. The ultimate solution is to have a very strict policy, with sophisticated testing procedures (that are strongly enforced at a low cost), almost taking a "guilty until proven innocent" approach. However, athletes' rights could be violated and the process could lead to drawn-out court battles and lawsuits, ultimately rendering the testing useless.

Testing for steroids is done via measurement of the athletes' urine samples using technologies such as gas (and liquid) chromatography-mass spectrometry and high-resolution mass spectrometry (although other methods are being explored). Anabolic steroid metabolites found in the urine indicate a failed drug test. For detection of testosterone use, the ratio of testosterone found in the urine to its metabolite epitestosterone (T:E ratio) is a common marker. Historically, a ratio of 6:1 was used, but that has been lowered to 4:1. A test showing a ratio larger than this indicates testosterone use. A ratio of 1:1 is normal for most individuals. Therefore, a ratio of 6:1— and now 4:1—was arbitrarily set, though it still enabled the athletes to use testosterone or other drugs known to increase endogenous testosterone. However, athletes are known to "beat" drug testing using several techniques, including diluting urine volume, contaminating urine samples, using masking agents (many of which are banned), gradually cycling down or discontinuing steroid use when the testing date is known, using steroids with shorter detection times, consuming epitestosterone to balance the T:E ratio, and substituting another urine sample for their own. Although undocumented, it does appear that many athletes are aware of these practices, which undoubtedly have resulted in very low numbers of steroid-using athletes testing positive.

Human Growth Hormone

Human growth hormone (HGH) is released from the anterior pituitary and has several anabolic, fat-burning, and performance-enhancing functions similar to testosterone. The anabolic properties stimulate growth in bone and skeletal muscle, but also affect other major organs, leading to potential side effects. Other biologically potent isoforms of HGH exist, and these appear to be suppressed by HGH use as well. HGH is naturally secreted in pulsatile bursts (i.e., large amounts are secreted during fixed intervals), mostly during sleep, and HGH is the most responsive anabolic hormone to the acute stress of high-intensity exercise. Many of the HGH effects are mediated by another protein hormone, insulin-like growth factor-1 (IGF-1). Upon secretion into circulation, HGH binds to receptors on the liver and increases the secretion of IGF-1, which is thought to mediate many of the anabolic actions. IGF-1 is another hormone/drug used by athletes.

Recombinant HGH has been used clinically to treat several ailments. However, athletes have been aware of HGH's anabolic potential since the late 1980s and HGH has been used and abused by athletes ever since, with some indication that use is much higher now than 10 years ago. Not only can strength and power athletes benefit from HGH, but it was recently shown that HGH exerts potent anabolic effects in endurance runners. Another important aspect of HGH is its role in enhancing connective-tissue strength. This effect leads some athletes to use HGH to counteract the potential damaging effects of anabolic steroids on tendons. Taking HGH is thought to reduce the potential for injury that is increased with the use of steroids, while still providing an anabolic effect.

Interestingly, some studies have indicated that the effects of HGH alone on skeletal muscle may not be that potent. However, many of those studies examined nonathletes (e.g., the elderly) using clinical doses. Most athletes who use HGH (at doses far exceeding clinical recommendations) attest to benefiting greatly from it. Although HGH by itself is ergogenic, it is believed that the largest effects are seen when HGH is stacked with anabolic steroids (and possibly other anabolic agents). The synergistic effect of the two is thought to provide greater anabolic potency than either one alone. In fact, the synergistic effect of HGH and anabolic steroids was shown in regards to cardiac muscle hypertrophy, where the addition of HGH to anabolic steroid use led to higher left ventricular mass.

HGH is extremely expensive. Even on the black market, the cost of HGH far exceeds that of anabolic steroids, meaning that athletes with higher incomes or resources are most likely to use HGH. Humatrope, Nutropin, Norditropin, Genotropin, Serostim, Saizen, and Protropin can cost several thousand dollars per year. In fact, some professional bodybuilders have attested to spending $40,000 to $60,000 per year on drugs and supplements, with a substantial portion of that cost attributed to HGH. Some reports indicate that a dose of HGH can cost around $150 to $170 and a typical black market price is approximately $20 to $30 per IU. In addition, some athletes (mostly bodybuilders) have been reported to use about 0.3 IU per week for each pound of body weight, injected subcutaneously in small intervals. In fact, some high-level bodybuilders have used 6 to 12 IU per day in combination with anabolic steroids, thyroid hormones (T3), and insulin.

Human growth hormone is a protein molecule. Therefore, HGH is injected, because it would be digested if taken orally. Also, because it is a protein, it is not found in the urine (i.e., very little to no protein is found in urine in healthy individuals). Therefore, HGH cannot be detected in urine via drug testing. In fact, many athletes use HGH to escape detection. Other methods of determining HGH have been proposed and tested, including blood testing and measuring other secratogues, IGF-1, and other proteins. However, the current lack of detection is attractive to athletes competing at a high level.

The use of HGH can lead to significant side effects. These side effects are summarized in Figure 11-4. Some of these side effects lead to visual growth patterns (i.e., *acromegaly*) of bones which demonstrate HGH use. Coaches, growth in the bones in the forehead, jaw, hands, and feet are distinguishing features indicating HGH use in the athlete. Despite athletes vehemently denying HGH use, their appearance tells a different story, one that cannot be explained by training alone.

- Acromegaly (i.e. enlargement of the bones of the head, feet, and hands)
- Altered hormonal profiles
- Increased possibility of insulin resistance and diabetes
- Distended abdomen (from visceral tissue enlargement)
- Hypoglycemia (low blood sugar)
- Altered thyroid function
- High blood pressure
- Enlargement of the heart and lungs
- Impaired liver and muscle glycogen
- Potential kidney and liver damage
- Headaches
- Mood swings
- Menstrual disturbances

Figure 11-4. Side effects from human growth hormone use in athletes

Insulin

Insulin is a very potent anabolic hormone that is secreted by the pancreas in response to elevations in blood glucose and amino-acid concentrations. Insulin is involved in transporting glucose and amino acids into muscle cells, where protein synthesis occurs. In addition, insulin reduces fat breakdown and encourages fat storage. Like HGH, insulin is a protein hormone and is therefore is not present in urine. Because of its anabolic properties, athletes (who are not diabetic) have used insulin (i.e., Humulin-R, N, or L). Bodybuilders have used this drug to increase muscle size (although use among non-bodybuilders is on the rise), as some feel it potentiates the effects of HGH and IGF-1. Many bodybuilders have taken approximately 15 to 60 IU (or 1 IU for every 20 pounds of body weight) of insulin per day (i.e., 5 to 15 IU two to four times per day). In addition, many bodybuilders take large doses right after a workout. Some bodybuilders also take about 10 grams of carbohydrates for every IU of insulin approximately 30 minutes following insulin injection. A major side effect of insulin use is hypoglycemia (i.e., low blood sugar), which could be fatal. Therefore, insulin use can be very dangerous and is highly ill-advised.

Insulin-Like Growth Factor-1 (IGF-1)

Many of the anabolic effects of HGH are mediated by IGF-1. Therefore, similar benefits are sought by athletes who take IGF-1. IGF-1 is also very costly and is thought to produce side effects similar to those of HGH. As a protein, IGF-1 is not detectable in urine, although other methods of assessment are being explored.

Human Chorionic Gonadotropin (HCG)

HCG is a glycoprotein hormone found in the placenta of women. Some athletes use HCG because it has been shown to stimulate the Leydig cells to produce testosterone naturally. In fact, a dose of 3000 IU of HCG has been shown to result in significant elevations in testosterone in athletes. HCG is often stacked with anabolic steroids, especially when athletes are cycling down. Stacking with HCG is thought to allow athletes to rejuvenate their testicular size and increase the testosterone-producing capacity that becomes limited during steroid use. Stacking HCG also assists in the maintenance of some of the anabolic effects associated with anabolic steroids. In addition, HCG is thought to increase natural testosterone production and stabilize the T:E ratio for athletes doping with testosterone (as it increases both testosterone and epitestosterone in urine). Because HCG increases testosterone, several of the side effects seen with testosterone or anabolic steroid use may also be seen with HCG, especially at higher doses. Doses of 1000 to 7000 IU of HCG injected every five days have been used by athletes in three- to four-week cycles, although some athletes have reportedly used greater quantities for cycles extending beyond eight weeks.

Clenbuterol

Clenbuterol (brands names include Spiropent, Prontovent, Novegam, Clenasma, and Broncoterol) is a drug classified as a β2 agonist, meaning that it is similar to drugs such as albuterol, salmeterol, and bromobuterol. Generally, β2 agonists have been used to treat asthma because they cause bronchodilation, which acts as a respiratory aid. In addition, β2 agonists induce other hormonal, metabolic, cardiovascular, and sympathetic nervous system stimulant effects associated with an "adrenaline response," as seen with ephedrine. Clenbuterol, while banned in the United States, has been used to treat asthma in other countries. However, many athletes have used clenbuterol because it has been shown to have two significant ergogenic effects. It has been shown to increase muscle mass (mostly by reducing protein breakdown, especially in fast-twitch fibers) and strength (more so than other β2 agonists). In addition, clenbuterol increases lipolysis, the body's fat-burning (thermogenic) ability. This body fat–reducing component is attractive to athletes who are maintaining weight or striving to improve appearance. In some cases, clenbuterol can reverse some of the lipogenic effects of insulin for those athletes using that drug to enhance muscle size. Some studies have shown clenbuterol can enhance muscle strength and power in humans. Clenbuterol and other β2 agonists have been used to increase lean tissue in the livestock industry.

Clenbuterol is often stacked with other drugs when used by athletes. It has also been used in an "on/off" manner, meaning that athletes will use it for two to three weeks at doses of approximately 60 to 140 micrograms per day (or three to seven tablets taken in divided doses each day) and then discontinue use for two to three weeks. Among athletes, clenbuterol tends to be viewed as an effective short-term drug due to the fact that receptor downregulation can take place quickly, thereby limiting the ergogenic effects in the long term. Many athletes have preferred to consume clenbuterol in tablet form rather than use the spray form. In addition, clenbuterol is commonly stacked with anabolic steroids and used during "off" steroid cycles to maintain lean-tissue mass prior to the initiation of a new steroid cycle.

The half-life of clenbuterol is approximately 35 hours and it accumulates with subsequent repeated doses. Approximately 97 percent of clenbuterol is removed from the body within eight days. Therefore, a failed drug test can result during this time. Although clenbuterol has been touted as a "safe alternative to steroid use," it does have significant side effects. Reports of increased heart rate, increases in the heart's force of contraction, tremors, muscle cramps, palpitations, insomnia, nervousness, and headaches have been documented. In addition, clenbuterol may result in greater excretion of minerals (e.g., potassium, magnesium), which can be dangerous when this drug is taken in tandem with diuretics (as some bodybuilders do).

Coaching Points

All of the anabolic agents discussed in this chapter are banned substances unless they are being used for medicinal purposes. Therefore, steep punishments may be faced if an athlete tests positive for a banned substance or is found possessing these anabolic agents. While all of these agents are ergogenic, coaches should monitor athletes closely for drug use. Being naïve, pleading ignorance, or taking a "blind eye" approach (i.e., thinking a problem exists but having no willingness to deal with it) will not curtail anabolic steroid use, especially among young athletes. With all of the potential ergogenic effects seen with these drugs, the willingness to experiment is at an all-time high, especially if young athletes believe their performance will be enhanced and the possibility to compete at a higher level exists. Because athletes are not likely to disclose anabolic drug use to most individuals (especially coaches), you should look for some general signs of drug use and persistently question an athlete if several of the following factors are observed. Although many side effects have already been discussed, the following list includes visible factors that the coach should be able to identify:

- A substantial increase in muscle mass or strength is seen in a relatively short period of time (or a loss of significant mass and strength resulting from coming off a cycle).

- The athlete develops significant unexplainable acne, a rash, an increase in body hair, or clammy skin.

- Acromegaly, or bone growth, is present, especially in the head, face, hands, and feet (indicating potential HGH or IGF-1 use)

- Gynecomastia (breast development) occurs.

- A change in temperament, mood swings, or a sudden increase in aggressive behavior is seen.

- In young athletes, watch for increased muscle mass that appears disproportionate with body structure, which is a sign that some premature growth-plate closure has taken place in the skeletal system from the use of anabolic steroids.

- Masculinization and bloating appear in the face, giving the athlete the appearance of aggression (or anger) in his facial expression

- Signs of steroid use are present (e.g., steroid-related information, needles, vials, pill bottles). Also, be wary of athletes associating with known steroid users or distributors.

12

Blood Doping and Erythropoietin

Blood doping, or blood boosting, refers to the infusion of blood or blood products to increase athletic performance. The use of blood doping in sports is thought to date back to the early 1960s, when an elite cyclist was alleged to have used this technique in Tour de France competition. Other reports surfaced of endurance athletes using this technique during the 1972 Olympic Games. Since then, endurance athletes (e.g., cyclists, cross-country skiers, distance runners, triathletes) have predominantly used blood doping to enhance endurance performance. Although this technique was banned by the International Olympic Committee (IOC) in 1984, the drug *erythropoietin* (EPO) became the method of choice to "boost blood" in 1988. Other erythropoiesis- (red blood cell formation) or EPO-enhancing agents (e.g., *darbepoietin-α*) have been examined, as has gene therapy.

Before examining the physiological effects of blood doping, it is important to understand the process of oxygen transport and delivery in the human body. Oxygen travels through arterial blood (that is oxygenated in the lungs) until it reaches the target tissue. *Red blood cells* (i.e., erythrocytes) transport oxygen and contain *hemoglobin*, an iron-containing protein that carries oxygen. A gram of hemoglobin carries approximately 1.34 milliliters of oxygen. Hemoglobin is a potent acid-base buffer that also has implications for enhancing anaerobic-exercise performance. Typical values of hemoglobin in men and women are 14 to 18 and 12 to 16 grams per deciliter of blood, respectively. Therefore, an athlete could improve his oxygen-carrying capacity (and $\dot{V}O_2$ max) by increasing red blood cell count and hemoglobin concentrations. This process can be done naturally through aerobic training, especially at high altitudes (or just by living at altitude). However, it can also be done via blood doping and erythropoietin use.

The technique for blood doping involves intravenous injection of blood into the body. The blood may come from a donor (this is called homologous infusion), but most times the athlete will have his own blood withdrawn over the course of weeks (this is called autologous infusion), frozen in glycerol (to reduce hemolysis), and reinfused three to five days before a competition (after the red blood cells are washed with saline). The goal is to increase the body's oxygen-carrying capacity. This technique has been shown to increase red blood cell content by an average of up to 10 percent. One to four units (450 to 1800 milliliters) are withdrawn and spun (i.e., centrifuged). The process of centrifugation separates blood into plasma (i.e., the liquid portion) and packed cell content. The packed red blood cell content is typically frozen for eight to 12 weeks before competition, as this amount of time is needed for the body to regain its own red blood cell count and hemoglobin content. The typical lifetime of a red blood cell lasts approximately 120 days. However, this timeframe is shorter in endurance athletes due to the stress of rigorous training and competition. Therefore, it takes longer to completely recover from blood withdrawal during endurance training. These athletes may experience some fatigue or the effects of detraining during the time of blood extraction.

Ergogenic Effects

Research has shown that blood doping can enhance performance, and the effects of blood doping can be seen within 24 hours of blood infusion. The intent behind blood doping is to increase red blood cell content and hemoglobin concentrations. By doing so, $\dot{V}O_2$ max, buffer capacity, thermoregulation (i.e., heat tolerance), and subsequent endurance performance can significantly increase. Although blood volume also increases, the majority of the ergogenic effects associated with blood doping are due to the oxygen availability/transport effects seen with higher red blood cell counts and hemoglobin concentrations. These ergogenic effects may persist for several weeks, although a gradual reduction takes place as time goes by.

The ergogenic effects of blood doping were first shown in 1947 when Pace and colleagues reinfused 2 liters of whole blood and found enhanced performance. Since then, numerous studies using either infusion of 1000 to 1200 milliliters of whole blood or 400 to 500 milliliters of packed red blood cells have shown ergogenic effects. Note that research has shown that both infusion methods produce similar ergogenic effects. Blood doping has been shown to increase $\dot{V}O_2$ max by up to 11 percent, 5-mile treadmill run time, 10-kilometer race time, and running and cycling time to exhaustion by 13 to 26 percent. In addition, Sawka and colleagues (1987) showed that VO_2 max increases from blood doping were greater in those athletes with high levels of aerobic fitness ($\dot{V}O_2$ max greater than 50 milliliters per kilogram of body mass per minute). The majority of ergogenic effects are seen at sea level. Some to most of the ergogenic effects are lost when performing exercise at high altitudes.

Side Effects

Because blood doping is more transient in nature, side effects typically include problems associated with the blood draw/transfusion process or from having too high of a blood volume. Hyperviscosity of blood increases vascular resistance, which can increase the likelihood of a stroke or other cardiovascular event. Viscous blood decreases peripheral flow and cardiac output, thereby reducing aerobic capacity. Complications can occur from the infusion process, such as allergic reactions and bacterial/viral infections. In addition, mislabeling or improper handling of blood can lead to more severe illnesses.

Erythropoietin (EPO)

Erythropoietin (EPO) is a glycoprotein hormone produced by the kidneys and liver that stimulates the production of red blood cells (a process known as erythropoiesis). Oxygen availability in the kidneys and liver is an important regulator of EPO production. Therefore, hypoxia (i.e., a lack of oxygen) leads to greater synthesis and secretion of EPO, which is why living and/or training at altitude increases concentrations of EPO. Remember, hypoxia occurs naturally at high altitudes due to the lower partial pressure of oxygen. When EPO is released into circulation it binds to receptors in bone marrow, which ultimately stimulates greater red blood cell production. A large variability exists in the secretion of this hormone, thereby making it difficult to test for EPO use among endurance athletes.

The synthetic form of EPO is recombinant human EPO (rhEPO), which has great clinical relevance, especially for treating anemia and other severe illnesses. Because it is a glycoprotein, rhEPO is injected into the blood (or subcutaneously) to increase red blood cell counts and hemoglobin concentrations. rhEPO cannot be readily distinguished from normal EPO produced by the body. Repeated injections of EPO will increase hemoglobin concentration in a dose- and time-dependent manner. Studies have shown that three to seven weeks of rhEPO (20 to 50 IU per kilogram of body mass three times per week) increased hemoglobin by approximately 6 to 11 percent, $\dot{V}O_2$ max by 7 percent, and hematocrit by 6 to 8.3 percent. Three to seven weeks of rhEPO at these same doses decreased blood lactate during exercise and run time to exhaustion by 17 percent. In fact, five weeks of lower doses of rhEPO (20 IU per kilogram of body mass) was effective for maintaining a 6 to 8 percent increase in $\dot{V}O_2$ max that followed three weeks of higher dose rhEPO use (50 IU per kilogram of body mass).

Doping with EPO (along with iron supplementation) must be done weeks or even months prior to major competitions to enhance training and competition performance. When rhEPO is injected intravenously, peak blood values occur quickly and the half-life is approximately four to five hours. When injected subcutaneously, rhEPO takes approximately 12 to 18 hours to peak and the half-life increases to up to 24 hours. The use of EPO may pose some similar risks to blood doping. Increases in blood pressure and flu-like symptoms have been observed with EPO use.

Drug Testing and Detection

Because EPO is a protein, urine testing was not sufficient to detect doping until technological advances alleviated the problem. Blood testing had been viewed as an alternative. However, blood detection has its own set of problems. Individual variation can explain substantial elevations in EPO, especially after exposure to altitude, stress, or dehydration. In addition, the duration of the ergogenic effects of rhEPO use is greater than the detection period, meaning that an athlete may not produce a positive test but may still be benefiting from prior rhEPO use. In fact, Russell and colleagues (2002) found $\dot{V}O_2$ max to be elevated one month after rhEPO administration.

The presence of rhEPO in both blood and urine can be detected, as rhEPO produces a less negative charge than EPO produced in the body. In fact, detection of rhEPO in 100 percent of cases is seen if performed within 24 hours of use and in 75 percent of athletes if performed after 48 hours of use. Measuring EPO levels in the blood has been suggested as a possible test method. Use of rhEPO has been shown to increase blood EPO concentrations threefold. However, blood levels can return to their baseline values 48 to 72 hours after the last injection.

Other indirect indicators of rhEPO use have been proposed to determine current as well as prior use. These indicators are markers of abnormal or excessive red blood cell formation. Some of these methods include examining the following:

- The level of soluble transferrin receptors (sTfR) in the blood (which may double), as well as the ratio of sTfR to ferritin

- Hematocrit levels

- The percentage of reticulocytes (immature red blood cells that have shed their nucleus)—a useful indicator of erythropoiesis

- Percentage of macrocytes (large red blood cells indicative of reticulocyte formation)

International sport-governing bodies have provided their own standards. For example, the International Cycling Union has established hematocrit values of less than 47 and 50 percent for women and men, respectively, as acceptable for competition. The International Skiing Federation has established a hemoglobin level of 18.5 grams per 100 milliliters of blood (equating to a hematocrit of approximately 56 percent). In a study by Birkeland and colleagues (2000), endurance athletes were given 5000 units of rhEPO three times per week and every subject in the study had a hematocrit increase to at least 50 percent.

Coaching Points

- Although blood doping and the use of rhEPO can improve athletic performance, especially in those activities that rely on endurance, blood-boosting techniques are banned by the IOC and are unethical for all athletes.

- Blood-boosting techniques have an inherent risk of increasing blood viscosity, which could lead to potential cardiovascular problems.

- Coaches should be aware of the acute effects mentioned in this chapter and closely monitor athletes for doping.

- Substantial increases in $\dot{V}O_2$ max and endurance performance in a very short period of time (that is not indicative of training variation) should encourage you to question the athlete about the potential use of blood-boosting techniques.

13

Stimulants, Recreational Drugs, and Other Ergogenic Drugs

Stimulants, which are sympathomimetic agents, provide a boost to the central nervous system (CNS). Stimulants include amphetamines, caffeine, ephedrine (refer to Chapter 9), and cocaine (Figure 13-1). Each stimulant has its own characteristic mechanism of action on CNS neurons and their associated receptors and nerve terminals. Stimulants share common physiological effects. Figure 13-2 lists these potential ergogenic effects, while Figure 13-3 lists some of the many side effects associated with the use of stimulants. Athletes looking to gain an advantage use stimulants for these "fight or flight" responses, which mimic the actions of the sympathetic nervous system. The use of stimulants can lead to acute increases in strength, endurance, and power, and improvements in performance can also be seen. The thermogenic effects help with weight control and body-fat loss. Other drugs commonly used by athletes include diuretics, anti-estrogens, thyroid hormones, masking agents, and various recreational drugs.

Amphetamines

Amphetamines (i.e., "speed") were first synthesized in 1887, but were not medically used until 1927. When athletes began experimenting with amphetamines is unclear, but the American Medical Association, in conjunction with the NCAA, began investigating alleged widespread use of amphetamines by athletes in 1957. Amphetamines are banned substances, but they are still used by athletes to improve performance. A report focusing on collegiate hockey players showed that 7 to 16 percent reported some past or present use of amphetamines (Bents et al., 2004). In fact, a NCAA-published report indicates that amphetamine use has been on the rise in college sports since 1997, although athletes claim the rationale for use was social and personal, not ergogenic. Most athletes reported that the sources of amphetamines were friends or relatives.

Amphetamines release stores of norepinephrine, serotonin, and dopamine from nerve endings, and prevent reuptake, which leads to greater amounts of dopamine and norepinephrine in synaptic clefts. The sympathetic response is greatly enhanced by greater neurotransmitter availability. Amphetamines, which are typically ingested orally, injected, smoked, or snorted, are absorbed from the small intestine. Peak blood concentrations occur one to two hours following use. Effects may be seen within 10 to 40 minutes of consumption and may last up to six hours. Amphetamine metabolites are excreted in the urine, where they can be detected (for up to four days following use) via drug testing. Lastly, amphetamines are very addictive, so athletes should be

- Adrafinil
- Amfepramone
- Amiphenazole
- Amphetaminil
- Benzphetamine
- Bromantan
- Carphedon
- Cathine
- Clobenzorex
- Cocaine
- Dimethylamphetamine
- Ephedrine
- Etilamphetamine
- Etilefrine
- Famprofazone
- Fencamfamin
- Fencamine
- Fenetylline
- Fenfluramine
- Fenproporex
- Furfenorex

- Mefenorex
- Mephentermine
- Mesocarb
- Methamphetamine
- Methylamphetamine
- Methylenedioxyamphetamine
- Methylenedioxymethamphetamine
- Methylephedrine
- Methylphenidate
- Modafinil
- Nikethamide
- Norfenfluramine
- Parahydroxyamphetamine
- Pemoline
- Phendimetrazine
- Phenmetrazine
- Phentermine
- Prolintane
- Selegiline
- Strychnine

Figure 13-1. List of banned stimulants

very concerned, as a "harmless experiment" can easily turn into an addictive habit. Once tolerance is built to the drug, the user falls into the trap of using more and more to get the desired effects. In this scenario, addiction and potential side effects are far more likely.

- Increased heart rate
- Increased lipolysis and fat burning
- Increased blood pressure
- Suppressed appetite
- Increased breathing rate
- Greater arousal and alertness
- Increased metabolic rate and energy
- Increased endurance and time to exhaustion
- Greater concentration
- Greater speed and power
- Increased peak torque
- Elevation in catecholamines (adrenaline)
- Higher blood lactates
- Euphoria
- Aggression

Figure 13-2. Physiological effects of stimulants

- Tachycardia (chronic high heart rate)
- Heart palpitations
- Chronic elevation in blood pressure
- Cardiomyopathy
- Coronary heart disease and enlarged heart
- Restlessness
- Dizziness
- Insomnia
- Tremors
- Headaches
- Increased risk of stroke
- Increased risk of heart attack
- Muscle aches/cramps
- Impulsive behavior
- Loss of coordination (long-term use)
- Dryness of mouth
- Dehydration
- Gastrointestinal distress
- Diarrhea or constipation
- Aortic abnormalities
- Possibly anorexia nervosa
- Anxiety and irritability
- Greater perspiration
- Feelings of paranoia
- Psychosis (heavy use)
- Menstrual irregularities
- Depression
- Hallucinations
- Brain damage (long-term use)

Figure 13-3. Side effects of stimulant use

Caffeine

Caffeine is one of the world's most widely used and accepted drugs. Pharmacologically, it is part of a group of stimulants called *methylxanthines*, or *xanthines*, which occur naturally in some plants, (e.g., coffee beans, tea leaves, cocoa leaves, and kola nuts). Caffeine is found and consumed legally in several products, including coffee (30 to 180 milligrams per serving), sodas (30 to 72 milligrams per serving), chocolate (2 to 35 milligrams per serving), and tea (25 to 110 milligrams per serving), and poses few serious side effects in comparison to other more potent stimulants (Figure 13-4).

Although caffeine is not a banned substance for athletes per se, an athlete could fail a drug test if his urinary levels exceed the established standard. Currently, levels above 12 micrograms per milliliter are banned by the International Olympic Committee (IOC) and above 15 micrograms per milliliter are banned from the NCAA. To exceed these levels a 150-pound athlete would have to drink approximately six cups of coffee or more (depending on the beverage's caffeine content) relatively quickly (within 20 to 30 minutes) and within two to three hours of testing. This amount of caffeine equates to approximately 9 grams per kilogram of body mass. It is not easy to reach this level of caffeine in the urine, as only up to 3 percent of orally ingested caffeine reaches the urine (the rest is metabolized to other by-products). In most cases, a urine sample in excess of these amounts suggests that the athlete has deliberately taken caffeine in capsule or tablet form with the intent of enhancing performance. Caffeine may be used as a legal ergogenic aid, provided that the dose does not exceed established limits.

Caffeine may enhance exercise performance by stimulating the CNS, which changes the perception of effort and/or muscle-fiber activation, affects calcium transport and enzymes controlling muscle glycogen, and increases fat breakdown via a higher adrenaline response. The increased fatty-acid availability increases fat oxidation and spares muscle glycogen. Research has shown that caffeine increases exercise performance (mostly endurance) by 20 to 50 percent with as little as 3 grams per kilogram of body mass. In fact, caffeine consumption of 250 to 330 milligrams, or 5 to 13 milligrams per kilogram of body mass, has been shown to increase running/cycling time to exhaustion and total work during exercise. During short-term, (four to 35 minutes) higher-intensity exercise, caffeine consumption has been shown to improve swim trials, rowing time trials, and run and cycle time to exhaustion. Short-term (30 to 90 seconds), high-intensity exercise is minimally affected by caffeine consumption. Some studies have shown no improvements in maximal cycling power. However, caffeine-plus-ephedrine has been shown to enhance anaerobic power and appears to provide a potent thermogenic effect. Trained athletes may respond better to caffeine consumption than untrained individuals.

Caffeine may slightly enhance muscle strength. Consumption of 3 to 6 grams of caffeine per kilogram of body mass results in urinary caffeine levels that fall well within

Soft Drink (12-oz. serving)	Caffeine content (mg)
Jolt®	72.0
Sugar-free Mr. Pibb®	58.8
Mountain Dew®	54.0
Coca-Cola® and Diet Coke®	45.6
Shasta® Cola	44.4
Dr. Pepper® and Diet Dr. Pepper®	39.6
Pepsi-Cola®	38.4
Diet Pepsi®	36.0
Sunkist® Orange Soda	40
7-Up® and Sprite®	0

Tea (5-ounce cup)	Caffeine content (mg)
1-minute brew	9–33
3-minute brew	20–46
5-minute brew	20–50
Instant tea	12–28
Iced tea (12-ounce cup)	22–36
Green tea	30
Snapple® iced tea (16-ounce)	48

Coffee (5-ounce cup)	Caffeine content (mg)
Drip method	110–150
Percolated	64–124
Instant	40–108
Decaffeinated	2–5
Instant decaffeinated	2
Häagen-Dazs® coffee ice cream (1 cup)	58

OTC Preparations	Caffeine content per tablet (mg)
Stimulants	
NoDoz® tablets	100
Vivarin® tablets	200
Pain Relievers	
Anacin®	32
Excedrin®	65
Midol®	32

Chocolate	Caffeine content (mg)
Hershey's® bar (1.5 ounce)	10
Hot chocolate (8 ounce)	5
Pudding (5 ounce)	7
Ice cream (1/2 cup)	2

Note: mg = milligrams

Figure 13-4. Caffeine content of various beverages, foods, and pills

the legal range, while doses of 9 grams per kilogram of body mass may result in a range exceeding IOC standards 25 percent of the time. Consumption of 13 grams per kilogram of body mass may result in an illegal range 67 percent of the time. Limited side effects are shown with doses at or below 6 grams per kilogram of body mass. Therefore, the recommended dosing range for increasing performance is 3 to 6 grams of caffeine per kilogram of body mass. Ergogenic effects have been shown within this range, minimal side effects have been observed, and athletes will not produce urine samples out of range of the legally established standards. It is important to note that caffeine also has a slight diuretic effect, so proper hydration with caffeine use is important.

Cocaine

Cocaine is a highly addictive drug derived from the *Erythroxylon coca* plant. It has powerful stimulant, thermogenic, and euphoric effects. Cocaine is injected, snorted, inhaled, or smoked, and the effects are seen relatively quickly after consumption. The effects may last 20 to 30 minutes or longer (45 to 90 minutes) if the cocaine is inhaled. The half-life of cocaine is 30 to 40 minutes and cocaine metabolites can be found in the urine up to six days following use. The use of recreational drugs such as cocaine outweighs the use of performance-enhancing drugs in some athletic circles. As the American College of Sports Medicine has stated, cocaine use in athletes increased dramatically in the 1980s (approximately 17% of athletes surveyed), but has fallen substantially since then.

Ironically, the death of a few prominent athletes due to acute cocaine use sparked interest in its potential use in athletics. In elite sport settings, especially in professional athletics, fame, fortune, free time, and feelings of invincibility increase the likelihood that an athlete may experiment with cocaine. Most reports show no ergogenic effects— or show reduced athletic performance (i.e., *ergolytic* effects)—with cocaine use. In fact, one study has shown that acute cocaine consumption resulted in lower $\dot{V}O_2$ max and maximal heart rates during exercise (Marques-Magallanes et al., 1997). Behavioral changes may also occur. For examples, athletes may become more aggressive, irritable, and volatile. Although some athletes feel their performance is enhanced, confusion often exists regarding actual performance because the euphoric effects of cocaine disrupt perception. Cocaine has many dangerous side effects. Of critical importance is the risk for sudden death via cardiovascular abnormalities. The IOC, United States Olympic Committee (USOC), NCAA, and professional sports organizations have all banned cocaine use. Coaches beware—cocaine use is addictive, illegal, and dangerous for athletes, and should be avoided at all costs.

Diuretics

Diuretics are prescription drugs that block sodium reabsorption in the kidneys, thereby inducing the loss of fluid as well as some other electrolytes in addition to sodium (i.e., potassium, calcium, magnesium) in the urine. Diuretics have been used to treat diseases such as hypertension, congestive heart failure, edema, kidney, and liver problems. Because some diuretics block sodium reabsorption in the loop of Henle in the kidneys, they are known as loop diuretics (i.e., furosemide, bumetanide, ethacrynic acid, torsemide). Diuretics that block sodium reabsorption at the distal tubule are known as thiazides (i.e., chlorthalidone, hydrochlorothiazide, indapamide, metolazone, trichlormethiazide, quinethazone). Potassium-sparing diuretics block potassium secretion (i.e., amiloride, triamterene, spironolactone). Other types of diuretics exist but are much less commonly used by athletes.

Diuretics induce fluid loss via urine and assist in weight loss. Reports have shown that diuretics may result in a body-weight reduction of 3 to 4 percent over 24 hours. That equate to 6 to 8 pounds of fluid loss for a 200-pound athlete. Athletes sometimes take diuretics to make weight in sports that utilize weight classes. They are taken before weigh-ins and then the athlete rehydrates to regain lost weight prior to competition. Since weigh-ins are usually performed a day or two before competition (although some governing bodies are now requiring weigh-ins closer to the event), athletes who use diuretics have ample time to rehydrate, which enables them to compete at a higher weight than the weight class allows.

In addition, diuretics have been used by athletes to reduce the concentration of drugs in their urine via rapid diuresis, which reduces the likelihood of detection of banned drugs in a urine test (e.g., anabolic steroid use is sometimes masked with diuretics). Diuretics are one of the most commonly abused drugs in sport. In fact, Benzi (1994) has reported that diuretics were the fourth most commonly used drug among athletes, behind only anabolic steroids, stimulants, and narcotics. Sports such as wrestling, boxing, gymnastics, weight lifting, judo, power lifting, and mixed martial arts rely heavily on either making weight or maintaining a high strength-to-mass ratio. The use of dehydration methods to lose weight in these sports has often been reported. In general, a combination of heat exposure, exercise, food and water restriction, self-induced vomiting, laxatives, and diuretics has been used to lose weight. Diuretics, coupled with strict dieting, could increase the likelihood, or exacerbate the effects, of anorexia nervosa.

Bodybuilding is a sport with a high incidence of diuretic use. For bodybuilders, the goal is to lose body water to enhance appearance and look more defined (i.e., create a "ripped" appearance). Diuretics are typically taken four to seven days prior to competition to excrete excess water. However, diuretics have been implicated as the major factor contributing to several deaths, as bodybuilders dehydrated themselves to fatally low levels. Furosemide is the most widely used diuretic drug in bodybuilding. It is powerful and acts very quickly. Some bodybuilders have been reported to consume 20 to 40 milligrams of furosemide (Lasix) per day for a week prior to competition. In addition, some bodybuilders have also taken potassium-sparing diuretics to conserve electrolytes and to reduce incidence of cramping and other undesirable side effects associated with furosemide.

Diuretics have been banned by the NCAA, IOC, USOC, and various professional organizations. Urine samples containing diuretic residues result in a failed drug test. Therefore, athletes using diuretics are doing so illicitly. As mentioned previously, diuretics are also sometimes used to mask the use of other banned substances (many times anabolic steroids). The overall concentrations of banned substances are substantially lower in diluted urine, possibly allowing an athlete to escape detection. Because many athletes were able to avoid failed drug tests due to the use of diuretics, diuretics themselves were added to the banned substances list. Since this change was made, some athletes have been caught using furosemide, presumably to mask other banned substances.

Diuretics are drugs used only in the short-term, because they lead to dehydration as well as many other serious side effects (Figure 13-5). Dehydration could have a negative effect on performance. Studies have shown that 40 to 126 milligrams of furosemide resulted in 2- to 4-percent losses in body weight, as well as subsequent reductions in cycling performance, $\dot{V}O_2$ max, muscle strength, and rates of force development. It appears that the degree of performance loss is related to the degree of dehydration. Interestingly, the degree of performance loss appears greater when the dehydration results from exercise in the heat as opposed to diuretic use.

• Frequent urination	• Increased perspiration and restlessness
• Diarrhea	• Dehydration and rapid weight loss
• Arrhythmia	• Joint pain
• Muscle weakness, fatigue, and drowsiness	• Numbness in the extremities
• Muscle cramps and soreness	• Loss of appetite, nausea, and possibly vomiting
• Dizziness and light-headedness	• Fever, chills, or cough
• Blurred vision	• Alterations in glucose and fat metabolism
• Restlessness	
• Skin rash	• Reduced muscle glycogen
• Confusion	• Possibly coma or death with severe dehydration
• Headache	

Figure 13-5. Side effects of diuretics

Aerobic exercise performance appears to be more adversely affected by dehydration than anaerobic exercise performance. Some studies have shown reductions in strength and power, but others have shown no performance decrement with mild dehydration. A study showed that 40 milligrams of furosemide (resulting in a 2.2 percent reduction in body weight) did not negatively affect 50-, 200-, or 400-meter sprint times or vertical jump height (Watson et al., 2005). Diuretic use can potentially reduce performance. However, much of this reduction may be eliminated by rehydrating prior to competition.

Anti-Estrogens

Anabolic steroids and prohormones consumed by athletes in high concentrations are partially aromatized into estrogens (e.g., estradiol, estrone). Some anabolic steroids have minimal aromatizing properties (e.g., Deca Durabolin), while others are more potent (e.g., Equipoise, Dianabol, Halotestin, testosterone), thereby enticing athletes to use anti-estrogens as part of the drug stack.

Anti-estrogens have been successfully used to treat various diseases (e.g., breast cancer and infertility). However, athletes may use them to counteract the side effects of anabolic steroids. Some athletes report greater ergogenic gains when low-aromatizing steroids are used with minimal to zero use of anti-estrogens. However, the estrogen-like side effects are reduced with anti-estrogens. Several unwanted side effects of steroid use (e.g., feminizing effects such as gynecomastia, bloating, and other health risks) are caused by aromatization into estradiol and other estrogens. These high estrogen levels suppress the body's testosterone production. Studies show substantial elevations in estrogen levels with steroid use. Therefore, athletes seeking to reduce or minimize these unwanted effects may take anti-estrogens. In addition, anti-estrogens help restore natural testosterone production when athletes cycle down, and eventually off, of anabolic steroids and may raise HDL levels (which are depressed with steroid use).

Two categories of anti-estrogens exist—*aromatase inhibitors* and *receptor blockers*. Aromatase inhibitors block the enzyme that catalyzes the conversion to estrogens (e.g., *Cytadren*, which is also thought to inhibit cortisol production, *Aromasin*, *Teslac*, and *Arimidex*). Aromasin is thought to be one of the most effective aromatase inhibitors, if not the most effective. Receptor blockers antagonize (or block) the estrogen receptor, and include *Clomid* (clomiphene citrate), *Nolvadex* (tamoxifen citrate), *Evista* (raloxifene), and *Cyclofenil*.

Clomid is a popular drug among male bodybuilders who take doses of 50 to 100 milligrams per day to stimulate the body's testosterone production. This drug is frequently used for four to six weeks (possibly stacked with HCG) upon termination of a steroid cycle. Nolvadex is a popular anti-estrogen used by athletes (at doses of approximately 10 to 30 milligrams per day). Cytadren is also popular, as athletes have reported use of 250 to 500 milligrams per day (although higher doses may be used for the cortisol-controlling effect). Cyclofenil has been used at approximately 400 to 600 milligrams per day for four to five weeks following a steroid cycle. Aromatase inhibitors, selective estrogen-receptor blockers, and other anti-estrogens such as Clomid are prescription drugs that are banned by some sport governing bodies, including the World Anti-Doping Agency (WADA).

Thyroid Drugs

The thyroid gland produces two key regulatory metabolic hormones, triiodothyronine (T3) and thyroxine (T4). Thyroid hormones increase basal metabolic rate (BMR), cardiovascular response to exercise, carbohydrate metabolism, and tissue growth, and stimulate the breakdown of fat for energy use. They are typically used to treat thyroid insufficiency, obesity, and other metabolic disorders. From an anabolic perspective, thyroid hormones work in synergy with other anabolic hormones to potentiate the growth response. Athletes, especially bodybuilders, have used thyroid drugs to enhance the anabolic growth processes. Bodybuilders use them specifically to increase BMR to burn fat and get "ripped" prior to a competition. Thyroid drugs are often stacked with clenbuterol.

The metabolic effects of thyroid drugs appear to offset some of the negative effects of strict dieting, such as a slower metabolism. One popular thyroid drug is *Cytomel* (T3). Athletes have taken Cytomel in cyclical doses ranging from 25 to 100 micrograms per day for up to six weeks. Cytomel is considered a potent thyroid drug. Many athletes opt to take *Triacana* (T3) or *Synthroid* (T4), which tend to be less potent. Synthroid has been consumed in cyclical doses of 25 to 400 micrograms per day and Triacana has been consumed in cyclical doses of approximately 10 to 14 0.35-milligram tablets per day for four to eight weeks.

Thyroid hormone use can be dangerous. Consuming too much, or an abrupt stoppage in use, can upset the body's hormonal system, as thyroid hormones mediate several responses controlling secretion of other hormones. Negative side effects occur when the levels consumed are above, or too far below, normal function. Thyroid hormones in high doses can lead to a loss of skeletal muscle. In addition, other side effects include heart palpitations, agitation, shortness of breath, irregular heartbeat, sweating, nausea, restlessness, headaches, and mental and metabolic disorders. Long-term high doses can result in thyroid deficiency. Thyroid hormones are prescription drugs used for medicinal purposes and are unethical for use to enhance athletic performance.

Masking Agents

Masking agents are not ergogenic drugs. However, they are used to produce negative drug testing results by masking or hiding the use of banned performance-enhancing drugs. For example, diuretics have been used to dilute urine and mask drug use. Another class of drugs, sulfonamides, decreases the excretion rate of various drugs. In many cases, *sulfonamides* are used to slow the excretion rate of anabolic steroid metabolites, thereby allowing the user to escape detection during testing. However, these drugs were more effective when drug testing was more primitive in its development. Advanced technology can detect anabolic steroids in the urine despite the use of sulfonamides. In addition, one commonly used sulfonamide, *probenecid*, has been added to the banned substances list. Probenecid was developed in the 1950s to reduce the excretion of penicillin. Detection of probenecid results in a failed drug test and possible suspension. Use of probenecid has declined dramatically among athletes.

Athletes have also used epitestosterone as a masking agent. Chapter 11 covered the use of the T:E ratio for detecting testosterone use in athletes. Using epitestosterone reduces the T:E ratio to within legal limits (i.e., a 4:1 ratio), despite the athlete doping with testosterone. Therefore, testosterone use can be masked with epitestosterone. Reports from athletes have indicated that epitestosterone injections one hour prior to testing have resulted in a "passed" drug test. Lastly, other masking procedures such as urine substitution and catheterization have been used by athletes. These procedures are banned and stricter enforcement policies have decreased their use among athletes.

Beta Blockers

Beta blockers, or beta adrenergic antagonists, are a class of drugs that antagonize the effects of catecholamines, or adrenaline. They typically have been used to treat individuals with cardiovascular ailments. Catecholamines elicit the "fight or flight" response in the human body that prepares an individual for the stress of exercise or competition. Beta blockers reduce heart rate, force of contraction, and blood pressure.

Beta blockers are classified as *selective* or *nonselective* based on the response initiated by binding to β1, β2, or both receptors. Some nonselective beta blockers include propranolol, sotalol, nadolol, and penbutolol. Selective β1 beta blockers include acebutolol, metoprolol, atenolol, and bisoprolol. In the sports world, beta blockers are used to reduce anxiety and tension, provide better neuromuscular control, and increase performance in events that require great precision and accuracy. Athletes involved in sports where accuracy is critical have been known to use beta blockers as an ergogenic aid. Beta blockers are banned by WADA for specific sports, including archery, shooting, sailing, billiards, skiing, pentathlon, synchronized swimming, diving, and gymnastics.

Narcotics

Narcotics are a class of drugs that relieve pain (i.e., narcosis), relieve coughing, and act as an anesthesia. The term *narcotics* describe opium and its derivatives, as well as the analgesic effect produced when interaction with its specific opioid receptor occurs in the CNS. The juices from the opium poppy seed (*Papaver somniferum*) are the source of narcotics. *Morphine* makes up approximately 10 percent of this mixture.

Many different pharmaceutical agents are narcotics. However, in legal terms in the United States, only those that are addictive are considered narcotics. These drugs may be consumed orally; by injections subcutaneously, intravenously, and intramuscularly; rectally; and transdermally. Side effects include respiratory depression, dizziness, light-headedness, feeling faint, drowsiness, nausea, vomiting, and constipation. When narcotics are used for extended periods, they become habit-forming and very addictive. This physical dependence leads to significant withdrawal side effects upon stoppage, which makes narcotics a difficult drug class to quit. Heroin accounts for 90 percent of the narcotic abuse in the United States. Figure 13-6 presents some of the other commonly used and abused narcotics.

Athletes have been known to take narcotics. In fact, Benzi (1994) reported that narcotics were the third most commonly used drug class behind anabolic steroids and stimulants. The rationale for athletic use is predominantly pain relief, although some athletes crave the associated euphoria. It is unclear how much narcotics can directly help with sports performance. In clinical populations, aerobic exercise performance and

• Alfentanyl	• Methadone (Dolophine)
• Buprenorphine	• Morphine
• Butorphanol	• Nalbuphine (Nubain)
• Codeine	• Oxycodone (Percodan, OxyContin)
• Dextromoramide	• Oxymorphone
• Heroin	• Pentazocine
• Fentanyl	• Pethidine
• Hydrocodone (Vicodin)	• Propoxyphene (Darvon)
• Hydromorphone	• Remifentanyl
• Levorphanol	• Sufentanyl
• Meperidine (Demerol)	

Figure 13-6. Examples of narcotic drugs

tolerance may be enhanced. Clearly, athletes with injuries or substantial pain can benefit from the associated pain relief. Narcotics have been used not only to allow athletes to compete while injured, but also to train harder through injuries.

Narcotics are often used in conjunction with anti-inflammatory medications such as *corticosteroids* (which are not anabolic steroids) and *nonsteroidal anti-inflammatory drugs (NSAID)* to reduce pain and inflammation. Some professional athletes have come forward and expressed publicly their addiction to narcotics, which often resulted from initial use meant to help them play through pain. It is important to note that masking pain could result in further, more serious injury. Use of narcotics should only occur under medical supervision. Coaches should be aware of the addictive qualities of these drugs and have the medical staff closely supervise players with injuries who are prescribed narcotics for pain.

Other Recreational Drugs

Recreational, or social, drugs are commonly used in today's society. The athletic world is no exception. Recreational drugs are not taken for ergogenic purposes per se. However, some of the relaxing effects entice athletes to use them to better deal with the rigors of competition, practice, and preparation. Although athletes have been known to take many types of recreational drugs (some of which are discussed elsewhere in this book), this section covers alcohol, marijuana, and Gamma-hydroxybutyric acid (GHB).

Alcohol

Alcohol use is widely accepted in our culture. Alcohol consumption can begin as early as middle school, extend through college, and is very common in professional sports. Studies examining alcohol consumption among athletes have shown some interesting results. Stainback and Cohen (2002) have summarized these findings as follows:

- Male adolescents who participated in athletics were far more likely to begin drinking than nonathletes.

- Among high school seniors, athletes drank more frequently than sedentary seniors and were more inclined to binge drink

- Male and female intercollegiate athletes drank more alcohol per week, binge drank more often, experienced more adverse consequences from alcohol consumption, and engaged in more risk-taking behaviors than nonathletes. Examples of risky behavior included riding as a passenger with a drunk driver, not using seat belts, and fighting. Athletes in contact sports were more likely to engage in these behaviors and males were more likely to do so than females.

In addition, a survey of 262 male professional athletes indicated that all had previous alcohol use and more than 90 percent reported alcohol consumption within the last 30 days. It is clear that alcohol has become commonplace in sports and that athletes are a population at risk for extensive alcohol consumption.

Athletes may drink alcohol because they wish to relax, socialize, reduce inhibitions, or cope with everyday stress. However, the use of alcohol decreases reaction time and fine muscle coordination, and impairs balance, speech, vision, and hearing. Alcohol is a diuretic that leads to fluid loss and dehydration. It also negatively affects the body's thermoregulatory and sleep processes. The feeling of disinhibition and reduced anxiety is accompanied by loss of motor coordination, decreased reaction time, and lack of balance, coordination, and judgment. Alcohol leads to hypoglycemia and lowers muscle glycogen, which in turn leads to premature fatigue during exercise. In addition, alcohol weakens the immune system, thereby making an athlete more susceptible to bacterial and viral infections.

Acute alcohol consumption may reduce muscle strength and power, jump height, sprint time, and muscle and cardiovascular endurance, depending on the amount of alcohol consumed, the time frame of consumption, and the response (or tolerance) of the athlete. The effects of alcohol consumption are felt the day after in the form of a hangover. Symptoms of a hangover include muscle weakness and fatigue, hypoglycemia, nausea and vomiting, dehydration, dry mouth, headache, bloodshot eyes, hormonal imbalances (i.e., testosterone suppression), sweating, sensitivity to light and noise, and tremors. Hangovers reduce cognitive performance and athletic performance by an average of 11 percent, and increase the risk of injury by more than 25 percent.

Long-term alcohol abuse leads to greater tolerance, nutritional deficiencies, and tissue damage to virtually all organs, leading to greater risk of cancer, liver disease, and cardiovascular disease. Alcoholics have a life expectancy 15 years shorter than the average individual. In addition, alcoholism increases the likelihood of depression, suicide, accidents (and possible career-ending injuries), crime, homicides, and death. Although infrequent, moderate alcohol consumption (i.e., less than 0.5 ounces of alcohol per 23 kilograms of body mass per day) poses minimal risk, athletes and coaches need to be aware of the negative consequences associated with longer-term, uncontrolled alcohol abuse. In-competition alcohol consumption is banned by WADA for sports such as billiards, archery, skiing, and automobile and motorcycle sports. Clearly, alcohol use has been a central factor in numerous sport-related tragedies.

Marijuana

Marijuana is the most frequently used illicit substance in the United States. In fact, approximately 97 million Americans ages 12 and older have tried marijuana at least once and approximately 26 million people report marijuana use in the past year. Marijuana comes from the plant Cannabis sativa, which contains cannabinoids. One cannabinoid is the psychoactive substance, *delta-9-tetrahydrocannabinol (THC)*, which is the most active substance in marijuana. THC enters the brain in seconds and the effects of marijuana on the CNS are evident within minutes. The major route of entry of marijuana is via smoking. Athletes ingest marijuana for the psychological "high," which causes relaxation and a sense of euphoria. This high is dose-related and can last for several hours. In addition, some reports indicate marijuana may have a pain-relieving effect, which is another potential reason for use by athletes. Nevertheless, marijuana use is physiologically and psychologically addictive and a one-time trial can result in a habit.

Marijuana use produces numerous negative side effects. High doses cause hallucinations, delusions, paranoia, changes in personality, loss of memory, redness of the eyes, increased appetite, reduced immune function, and anxiety. Cardiovascular effects such as increased heart rate, blood pressure, and risk of heart attack have been noted. Because marijuana is smoked, the risk of respiratory infections is increased, along with other symptoms seen in cigarette smoking, such as coughing, phlegm, runny nose, sore throat, wheezing, bronchitis, and a greater risk for lung cancer. Long-term users show a lack of motivation, decreased concentration, poor judgment, and memory loss. From a performance perspective, marijuana results in reduced work capacity, impaired hand-eye coordination and reaction time, reduced motor coordination, fatigue, and impaired concentration and accuracy. Marijuana has no ergogenic potential to enhance sports performance. In addition, the reduced motor coordination from marijuana use can compromise the athlete's safety during performance of complex skills or contact sports.

The half-life of THC in the blood is about 20 hours and it is rapidly metabolized by the liver to *11-nor-9-delta-9-hydroxytetrahydrocannabinol* (THC-COOH), which can be detected in the urine via drug testing. The half-life of THC-COOH is 50 hours or more and detection may take place two to three days after smoking just one marijuana cigarette. Daily users can fail drug tests several weeks following last use. As much as 30 percent of the metabolites can remain in the body for one week. Complete elimination may take up to one month. Marijuana is a banned substance by the IOC, WADA, NCAA, and other sport governing bodies (e.g., NFL, MLB). A positive drug test can result in suspension, fine, or other form of punishment.

Gamma-Hydroxybutyric Acid (GHB)

Gamma-hydroxybutyric acid (GHB) is a powerful CNS depressant. GHB is produced naturally by the body in small amounts, mostly in the brain. Its physiological function is unclear, though it is thought to cause sedation and general anesthetic effects, and is very addictive. Consumption of low doses (less than 1 gram) of GHB (consumed orally in an odorless, tasteless, colorless liquid form or as a white powder easily dissolvable in liquids) causes relaxation and reduced inhibitions. At stronger doses, GHB interferes with blood circulation, motor coordination, and balance. High doses, especially when coupled with alcohol and other drugs that augment the effects, can lead to nausea, vomiting, delusions, depression, vertigo, hallucinations, drowsiness, muscle stiffness, slowed heart rate, lowered blood pressure, and more serious and potentially fatal respiratory depression, seizures, unconsciousness, coma, and overdose.

The average dose of 1 to 5 grams takes effect in 15 to 30 minutes, and the effects may last from three to six hours. Because GHB is short-lasting, withdrawal symptoms may occur within one to six hours of the last dose, thereby leading to further use and potential addiction. Because of the sedative effects, GHB is used as a "date rape" drug that is given to incapacitate unsuspecting victims. This potential use is a key reason the drug and its analogs were classified as Schedule I controlled substances (i.e., drugs with high potential for abuse and without any accepted medical use) by Congress in 2000.

GHB was sold in health food stores as a performance-enhancing agent until the FDA banned it from OTC use in 1990. It was thought that GHB stimulated growth-hormone secretion and subsequently increased muscle growth. It was popular among bodybuilders and other athletes. These effects have never been substantiated, but lifters still continued to experiment with GHB and some metabolites. In addition, some athletes have used GHB as a sleep aid, but this has been shown to be hazardous, as some prominent athletes have collapsed and become severely ill. A few have even died in response. Most of the GHB used today is "home-grown," made in kitchens by mixing various chemical ingredients. GHB is clearly a drug that should be avoided at all costs, as no ergogenic effects exist and the side effects can be fatal.

Future Considerations

Drug use in sports is common and will continue to be prevalent as long as athletic performance is rewarded with lucrative contracts, scholarships, wins, media coverage, and notoriety. Sanctions against drug use in sports are very limited and athletes are far ahead of any testing procedures currently in place. Trends reveal that professional and collegiate athletes will continue to take performance-enhancing drugs (perhaps at a higher rate), and that this use may matriculate even further into the high school and middle school levels.

For the most part, very little can be done to dissuade athletes from using performance-enhancing drugs. Only a few have suffered through suspension or scrutiny in the public eye from failed drug tests, while many athletes continue to use drugs without fear of penalty. Athletes are aware that their competitors and teammates may be using performance-enhancing drugs, so the consensus rationale appears to be, "Is it cheating if many are doing it?" or, "How can I compete if I don't?" Another question arises to the young athlete: "How good could I be if I used these substances?" These difficult questions are something many athletes do not want to address, which is why performance-enhancing drugs are commonplace in some sports. The loser turns out to be the natural athlete who competes on his own abilities.

Sport-governing bodies need to strictly enforce antidoping measures, but current testing policies are flawed or limited in technology, making it difficult to detect drug use. Coupled with repeated litigation from athletes who test positive and the overall cost of drug testing, it may be simpler for sport-governing bodies to close their eyes to the situation and in some unfortunate instances, this does occur. Coaches must be aware of signs of performance-enhancing drug use and take a personal interest in the supplementation practices of their athletes. Drug use may be disguised in several ways, but many of the signs discussed in this book are visible. Therefore, coaches can benefit from identifying these signs in players they suspect of using performance-enhancing drugs.

Although several doping measures have been discussed, the future of ergogenics appears to promise the enhancement of athletic performance to an even greater extent. In fact, some experts have suggested that the future of athletic performance may be determined greatly by future performance-enhancing advances in technology. Since the initiation of the Human Genome Project in 1990, in which the DNA sequences of approximately 95 percent of all human genes (approximately 50,000 in total) have been determined, several advances seem imminent, including the use gene transfer therapy, stem cells, or genetic engineering to modify athletes' genes, increase the synthesis of anabolic hormones, growth factors, and erythropoietin, and treat injuries. One growth factor in particular is *myostatin*, which is a potent inhibitor of muscle growth. Animals lacking this gene express large muscularity. Therefore, genetic engineering to inhibit this gene could result in sizable strength and size gains. Ways to enhance drug delivery (and increase the potency of current drugs) are being investigated. In addition, designer drugs will continue to be developed that have the potential to go undetected for long periods of time, thereby making them attractive to athletes hoping to beat the system. Future methods of doping will initially complicate the drug-detection system. In reality, it appears that athletes in the future will continue to have options for staying "ahead of the game."

Coaching Points

- Amphetamines, caffeine, ephedrine, and cocaine are stimulants that may increase endurance, strength, power, and ultimately athletic performance. Other than low-to-moderate levels of caffeine, these stimulants are banned substances and should not be used by athletes.

- Diuretics induce fluid (weight) loss and may be used by athletes to make weight or mask other illegal substances in the urine. These substances are banned and should not be used by athletes.

- Anti-estrogens are drugs that reduce some of the side effects from anabolic steroids. These also require a prescription and should not be used by athletes.

- Thyroid drugs increase metabolism and may potentiate muscle growth. Likewise, these require a prescription and should not be used for nonmedicinal purposes by athletes.

- Beta-blockers reduce the cardiovascular response and are used by athletes in sports requiring fine neuromuscular control. These substances are banned and should not be used by athletes.

- Narcotics relieve pain, are very addictive, and should only be used under a doctor's supervision.

- Alcohol and marijuana are recreational drugs that may reduce stress. Although alcohol consumption is legal, performance is negatively affected and coaches need to use discretion in monitoring alcohol use by athletes. Marijuana is a banned substance and should not be used by athletes.

Suggested Readings

Acacio, B.D. et al. (2004). Pharmacokinetics of dehydroepiandrosterone and its metabolites after long-term daily oral administration to healthy young men. *Fertility and Sterility*, 81: 595–604.

Achten, J. & Jeukendrup, A.E. (2004). Optimizing fat oxidation through exercise and diet. *Nutrition*, 20: 716–727.

Allen, J.D. et al. (1998). Ginseng supplementation does not enhance healthy young adults' peak aerobic exercise performance. *Journal of the American College of Nutrition*, 17: 462–466.

American College of Sports Medicine (2000). Alcohol and athletic performance. April.

American College of Sports Medicine (2000). Cocaine abuse in sports. May.

American College of Sports Medicine, American Dietetic Association, & Dieticians of Canada (2000). Joint Position Stand: Nutrition and athletic performance. *Medicine and Science in Sports and Exercise*, 32: 2130–2145.

American College of Sports Medicine (1996). The use of blood doping as an ergogenic aid. *Medicine and Science in Sports and Exercise*, 28: i–viii.

Andrews, J.L. et al. (2003). Carbohydrate loading and supplementation in endurance-trained women runners. *Journal of Applied Physiology*, 95: 584–590.

Angus, D.J., M. Hargreaves, J. Dancey, & M.A. Febbraio. Effect of carbohydrate or carbohydrate plus medium-chain triglyceride ingestion on cycling time trial performance. *J. Appl. Physiol.* 88: 113-119, 2000.

Anthony, J.C., Anthony, T.G., & Layman, D.K. (1999). Leucine supplementation enhances skeletal muscle recovery in rats following exercise. *Journal of Nutrition*, 129: 1102–1106.

Antonio, J. & Stout, J.R. (2002). *Supplements for Strength-Power Athletes*. Champaign, IL: Human Kinetics.

Antonio, J., Sanders, M.S., & Van Gammeren, D. (2001). The effects of bovine colostrum supplementation on body composition and exercise performance in active men and women. *Nutrition*, 17: 243–247.

Antonio, J. & Street, C. (1999). Glutamine: A potentially useful supplement for athletes. *Canadian Journal of Applied Physiology*, 24: 1–14.

Antonio, J. et al. (2000). Effects of exercise training and amino-acid supplementation on body composition and physical performance in untrained women. *Nutrition*, 16: 1043–1046.

Antonio, J. et al. (2000). The effects of Tribulus terrestris on body composition and exercise performance in resistance-trained males. *International Journal of Sport Nutrition Exercise and Metabolism*, 10: 208–215.

Armstrong, L.E. (2002). *Diuretics. In: Performance-Enhancing Substances in Sport and Exercise* (M.S. Bahrke & C.E. Yesalis, Eds.). Champaign, IL: Human Kinetics, pp. 109–116.

Bahrke, M.S. & Morgan, W.H. (2000). Evaluation of the ergogenic properties of ginseng: An update. *Sports Medicine*, 29: 113–133.

Ballantyne, C.S. et al. (2000) The acute effects of androstenedione supplementation in healthy young males. *Canadian Journal of Applied Physiology*, 25: 68–78.

Barnett, C. et al. (1994). Effect of L-carnitine supplementation on muscle and blood carnitine content and lactate accumulation during high-intensity sprint cycling. *International Journal of Sport Nutrition*, 4: 280–288.

Barr, S.I. (1999) Effects of dehydration on exercise performance. *Canadian Journal of Applied Physiology*, 24: 164–172.

Bartee, R.T. et al. (2004). Predictors of dietary supplement use among adolescent athletes. *Pediatric Exercise Science*, 16: 250–264.

Beckham, S.G & Earnest, C.P. (2003). Four weeks of androstenedione supplementation diminishes the treatment response in middle aged men. *British Journal of Sports Medicine*, 37: 212–218.

Bell, D.G. & Jacobs, I. (1999). Combined caffeine and ephedrine ingestion improves run times of Canadian Forces Warrior Test. *Aviation, Space and Environmental Medicine*. 70 : 325–329.

Bell, D.G., Jacobs, I., & Ellerington, K. (2001). Effect of caffeine and ephedrine ingestion on anaerobic exercise performance. *Medicine and Science in Sports and Exercise*, 33: 1399–1403.

Bell, D.G., Jacobs, I., & Zamecnik, J. (1998). Effects of caffeine, ephedrine and their combination on time to exhaustion during high-intensity exercise. *European Journal of Applied Physiology*, 77: 427–433.

Bendahan, D. et al. (2002). Citrulline/malate promotes aerobic energy production in human exercising muscle. *British Journal of Sports Medicine*, 36: 282–289.

Bents, R.T., Tokish, J.M., & Goldberg, L. (2004). Ephedrine, pseudoephedrine, and amphetamine prevalence in college hockey players. *Physician and Sports Medicine*, 32.

Benzi, G. (1994). Pharmacoepidemiology of the drugs used in sports as doping agents. *Pharmacological Research*, 29: 13–26.

Berardi, J.M. & Ziegenfuss, T.N. (2003). Effects of ribose supplementation on repeated sprint performance in men. *Journal of Strength and Conditioning Research*, 17: 47–52.

Bergstrom, J. et al. (1967). Diet, muscle glycogen and physical performance. Acta *Physioligica Scandinavica*, 71: 140–150.

Bidzinska, B. et al. (1993). Effect of different chronic intermittent stressors and acetyl-L-carnitine on hypothalamic beta-endorphin and GnRH on plasma testosterone levels in male rats. *Neuroendocrinology*, 57: 985–990.

Biolo, G., Fleming, R.Y.D., & Wolfe, R.R. (1995). Physiologic hyperinsulinemia stimulates protein synthesis and enhances transport of selected amino acids in human skeletal muscle. *Journal of Clinical Investigation*, 95: 811–819.

Biolo, G. et al. (1999). Insulin action on muscle protein kinetics and amino acid transport during recovery after resistance exercise. *Diabetes*, 48: 949–957.

Biolo G. et al. (1997). An abundant supply of amino acids enhances the metabolic effect of exercise on muscle protein. *American Journal of Physiology: Endocrinology and Metabolism*, 273: E122–E129.

Birkeland, K. et al. (2000) Effect of rhEPO administration on serum levels of sTfR and cycling performance. *Medicine and Science in Sports and Exercise*, 32: 1238–1243.

Boirie, Y. et al. (1997). Slow and fast dietary proteins differently modulate postprandial protein accretion. *Proceedings of the National Academy of Science*, 94: 14930–14935.

Borsheim E. et al. (2002). Essential amino acids and muscle protein recovery from resistance exercise. *American Journal of Physiology: Endocrinology and Metabolism*, 283: E648–E657.

Braam, L.A. et al. (2003). Factors affecting bone loss in female endurance athletes: A two-year follow-up study. *American Journal of Sports Medicine*, 31: 889–895.

Brault, J.J., Abraham, K.A., & Terjung, R.L. (2003). Muscle creatine uptake and creatine transporter expression in response to creatine supplementation and depletion. *Journal of Applied Physiology*, 94: 2173–2180.

Bredle, D.L. et al. (1988). Phosphate supplementation, cardiovascular function, and exercise performance in humans. *Journal of Applied Physiology*, 65: 1821–1826.

Brien, A.J. & Simon, T.L. (1987). The effects of red blood cell infusion on 10-km race time. *Journal of the American Medical Association*, 257: 2761–2765.

Brilla, L.R. & Conte, V. (2000). Effects of a novel zinc-magnesium formulation on hormones and strength. *Journal of Exercise Physiology*, 3: 26–36.

Brinkworth, G.D. et al. (2004). Effect of bovine colostrum supplementation on the composition of resistance trained and untrained limbs in healthy young men. European *Journal of Applied Physiology*, 91: 53–60.

Brinkworth, G.D. et al. (2002). Oral bovine colostrum supplementation enhances buffer capacity but not rowing performance in elite female rowers. *International Journal of Sport Nutrition and Exercise Metabolism*, 12: 349–365.

Britton, H.B. & Marshall, M.W. (1980). Effects of biotin, with or without sodium nitrate, on weight, food, fluid intake, and on methemoglobin, lactate, and lipids in the blood of rats. *Artery*, 7: 246–261.

Broeder, C.E. et al. (2000). The Andro Project: Physiological and hormonal influences of androstenedione supplementation in men 35 to 65 years old participating in a high-intensity resistance training program. *Archives of Internal Medicine*, 160: 3093–3104.

Brown, G.A., Vukovich, M.D., & King, D.S. (2004). Urinary excretion of steroid metabolites after chronic androstenedione ingestion. *Journal of Clinical Endocrinology and Metabolism*, 89: 6235–6238.

Brown, G.A. et al. (2004). Changes in serum testosterone and estradiol concentrations following acute androstenedione ingestion in young women. *Hormone and Metabolic Research*, 36: 62–66.

Brown, G.A. et al. (2002). Acute hormonal response to sublingual androstenediol intake in young men. *Journal of Applied Physiology*, 92: 142–146.

Brown, G.A. et al. (2001). Endocrine and lipid responses to chronic androstenediol-herbal supplementation in 30 to 58 year old men. *Journal of the American College of Nutrition*, 20: 520–528.

Brown, G.A. et al. (2000). Endocrine responses to chronic androstenedione intake in 30- to 56-year-old men. *Journal of Clinical Endocrinology and Metabolism*, 85: 4074–4080.

Brown, G.A. et al. (1999). Effect of oral DHEA on serum testosterone and adaptations to resistance training in young men. *Journal of Applied Physiology*, 87: 2274–2283.

Brown, R.C. & Cox, C.M. (1998). Effects of high fat versus high carbohydrate diets on plasma lipid and lipoproteins in endurance athletes. *Medicine and Science in Sports and Exercise*, 30: 1677–1683.

Brown, R.C., Cox, C.M., & Golding A. (2000). High-carbohydrate versus high-fat diets: Effect on body composition in trained cyclists. *Medicine and Science in Sports and Exercise*, 32: 690–694

Bucci, L.R. (2000). Selected herbals and human exercise performance. *American Journal of Clinical Nutrition,*. 72(suppl.): 624S–636S.

Buchman, A.L., Jenden D., & Roch, M. (1999). Plasma free, phospholipids-bound and urinary free choline all decrease during a marathon run and may be associated with impaired performance. *Journal of the American College of Nutrition*, 18: 598–601.

Buchman, A.L. et al. (2000). The effect of lecithin supplementation on plasma choline concentrations during a marathon. *Journal of the American College of Nutrition*, 19: 768–770.

Buckley, J.D., Brinksworth. G.D., & Abbott. M.J. (2003). Effect of bovine colostrum on anaerobic exercise performance and plasma insulin-like growth factor I. *Journal of Sport Science and Medicine*, 21: 577–588.

Buckley, J.D. et al. (2002). Bovine colostrum supplementation during endurance running training improves recovery, but not performance. *Journal of Sport Science and Medicine*, 5: 65–79.

Buick, F.J. et al. (1980). Effect of induced erythrocythemia on aerobic work capacity. *Journal of Applied Physiology*, 48: 636–642.

Burke, L.M. et al. (2000). Carbohydrate loading failed to improve 100-km cycling performance in a placebo-controlled trial. *Journal of Applied Physiology*, 88: 1284–1290.

Burns, R.D. et al. (2004). Intercollegiate student athlete use of nutritional supplements and the role of athletic trainers and dieticians in nutrition counseling. *Journal of the American Dietetic Association*, 104: 246–249.

Busquets, S. et al. (2002). Branched-chain amino acids: A role in skeletal muscle proteolysis in catabolic states? *Journal of Cell Physiology*, 191: 283–289.

Busquets, S. et al. (2000). Branched-chain amino acids inhibit proteolysis in rat skeletal muscle: Mechanisms involved. *Journal of Cell Physiology*, 184: 380–384.

Cabral de Oliveira, A.C. et al. (2005). Protection of Panax ginseng in injured muscles after eccentric exercise. *Journal of Ethnopharmacology*, 97: 211–214.

Cade, R. et al. (1984). Effects of phosphate loading on 2,3-diphosphoglycerate and maximal oxygen uptake. *Medicine and Science in Sports and Exercise*, 16: 263–268.

Candow, D.G. (2001). Effect of glutamine supplementation combined with resistance training in young adults. *European Journal of Applied Physiology*, 86: 142–149.

Castell, L.M. (2002). Can glutamine modify the apparent immunodepression observed after prolonged, exhaustive exercise? *Nutrition*, 18: 371–375.

Castell, L.M. & Newsholme, E.A. (1997). The effects of oral glutamine supplementation on athletes after prolonged, exhaustive exercise. *Nutrition*, 13: 738–742.

Catlin, D.H. et al. (2000). Trace contamination of over-the-counter androstenedione and positive urine test results for a nandrolone metabolite. *Journal of the American Medical Association*, 284: 2618–2621.

Chesley, A. et al. (1992). Changes in human muscle protein synthesis after resistance exercise. *Journal of Applied Physiology*, 73: 1383–1388.

Chester, N., Reilly T., & Mottram, D.R. (2003). Physiological, subjective and performance effects of pseudoephedrine and phenylpropanolamine during endurance running exercise. *International Journal of Sports Medicine*, 24: 3–8.

Chester, N. et al. (2004). Elimination of ephedrines in urine following multiple dosing: The consequences for athletes, in relation to doping control. *British Journal of Clinical Pharmacology*, 57: 62–67.

Chetlin, R.D. et al. (2000). The effect of ornithine alpha-ketoglutarate (OKG) on healthy, weight-trained men. *JEP Online*, 3: 37–47.

Chu, K.S. et al. (2002). A moderate dose of pseudoephedrine does not alter muscle contraction strength or anaerobic power. *Clinical Journal of Sports Medicine*, 12: 387–390.

Clancy, S.P. et al. (1994). Effects of chromium picolinate supplementation on body composition, strength, and urinary chromium loss in football players. *International Journal of Sport Nutrition*, 4: 142–153.

Clarkson, P.M. & Thompson, H.S. (2000). Antioxidants: What role do they play in physical activity and health? *American Journal of Clinical Nutrition*, 72 (suppl.): 637S–646S.

Collins, R.D. & Feldstein, A.H.. (2004). "Adulterated" androstenedione: What FDA's action against andro means for industry. *Sports Nutrition Review Journal*, 1: 52–60.

Collomp, K. et al. (1992). Benefits of caffeine ingestion on sprint performance in trained and untrained swimmers. *European Journal of Applied Physiology and Occupational Physiology*, 64: 377–380.

Colson, S.N. et al. (2005). Cordyceps sinensis- and Rhodiola rosea-based supplementation in male cyclists and its effect on muscle tissue oxygen saturation. *Journal of Strength and Conditioning Research*, 19: 358–363.

Connes, P. et al. (2004). Injections of recombinant human erythropoietin increases lactate influx into erythrocytes. *Journal of Applied Physiology*, 97: 326–332.

Connes, P. et al. (2003). Faster oxygen uptake kinetics at the onset of submaximal cycling exercise following 4 weeks recombinant human erythropoietin (r-HuEPO) treatment. *Pflugers Archives*, 447: 231–238.

Coombes, J.S. & Hamilton, K.L. The effectiveness of commercially available sport drinks. *Sports Medicine*, 29: 181–209.

Coombes, L.R. & McNaughton, L.R. (2000). Effects of branched-chain amino acid supplementation on serum creatine kinase and lactate dehydrogenase after prolonged exercise. *Journal of Sports Medicine and Physical Fitness*, 40: 240–246.

Coombes, J.S. et al. (2002). Dose effects of oral bovine colostrum on physical work capacity in cyclists. *Medince and Science in Sports and Exercise*, 34: 1184–1188.

Costill, D.L. et al. (1984). Acid-base balance during repeated bouts of exercise: Influence of HCO3. *International Journal of Sports Medicine*, 5: 228–231.

Cox, G. & Jenkins, D.G. (1994). The physiological and ventilatory responses to repeated 60-second sprints following sodium citrate ingestion. *Journal of Sports Science*, 12: 469–475.

Coyle, E.F. et al. (2001). Low-fat diet alters intramuscular substrates and reduces lipolysis and fat oxidation during exercise. *American Journal of Physiology: Endocrinology and Metabolism*, 280: E391–E398.

Craciun, A.M. et al. (1998). Improved bone metabolism in female athletes after vitamin K supplementation. *International Journal of Sports Medicine*, 19: 479–484.

Cynober, L. (1991). Ornithine alpha-ketoglutarate in nutritional support. *Nutrition*, 7: 313–322.

Daly, P.A. et al. (1993). Ephedrine, caffeine and aspirin: Safety and efficacy for treatment of human obesity. *International Journal of Obesity-Related Metabolic Disorders*, 17 (suppl.): S73–S78.

De Bock, K. et al. (2004). Acute Rhodiola rosea intake can improve endurance exercise performance. *International Journal of Sport Nutrition and Exercise Metabolism*, 14: 298–307.

Dietary Supplement Health and Education Act of 1994; Public Law 103-417, 103rd Congress. U.S. Food and Drug Administration.

Doessing, S. & Kjaer, M. (2005). Growth hormone and connective tissue in exercise. *Scandinavian Journal of Medicine and Science in Sports*, 15: 202–210.

Doherty, M. et al. (2002). Caffeine is ergogenic after supplementation of oral creatine monohydrate. *Medicine and Science in Sports and Exercise*, 34: 1785–1792.

Dowling, E.A. et al. (1996). Effect of Eleutherococcus senticosus on submaximal and maximal exercise performance. *Medicine and Science in Sports and Exercise*, 28: 482–489.

Duffy, D.J. & Conlee, R.K. (1986). Effects of phosphate loading on leg power and high-intensity treadmill exercise. *Medicine and Science in Sports and Exercise*, 18: 674–677.

Dunnett, M. & Harris, R.C. (1999). Influence of oral beta-alanine and L-histidine supplementation on the carnosine content of the gluteus medius. *Equine Veterinary Journal Supplement*, 30: 499–504.

Earnest, C.P. et al. (2004). Effects of a commercial herbal-based formula on exercise performance in cyclists. *Medicine and Science in Sports and Exercise*, 36: 504–509.

Earnest, C.P. et al. (2000). In vivo 4-androstene-3,17-dione and 4-androstene-3 beta,17 beta-diol supplementation in young men. *European Journal of Applied Physiology*, 81: 229–232.

Ekblom, B.T. (2002). *Erythropoietin. In: Performance-Enhancing Substances in Sport and Exercise* (Eds: M.S. Bahrke & C.E. Yesalis). Champaign, IL: Human Kinetics, pp. 101–108.

Embleton, P. & Thorne, G. (1998). *Musclemag International's Anabolic Primer*. Mississauga, ON: Musclemag International.

Engels, H.J. & Wirth, J.C. (1997). No ergogenic effects of ginseng (Panax ginseng C.A. Meyer) during graded maximal aerobic exercise. *Journal of the American Dietetic Association*, 97: 1110–1115.

Engels, H.J. et al. (2001). Effects of ginseng supplementation on supramaximal exercise performance and short-term recovery. *Journal of Strength and Conditioning Research*, 15: 290–295

Eschbach, L.F. et al. (2000). The effect of Siberian ginseng (Eleutherococcus senticosus) on substrate utilization and performance. *International Journal of Sport Nutrition and Exercise Metabolism*, 10: 444–451.

Evans, W.J. (2000). Vitamin E, vitamin C, and exercise. *American Journal of Clinical Nutrition*, 72 (suppl.): 647S–652S.

Farquhar, W.B. & Zambraski, E.J. (2002). Effects of creatine use on the athlete's kidney. *Current Sports Medicine Reports*, 1: 103–106.

Fawcett, J.P. et al. (1996). The effect of oral vanadyl sulfate on body composition and performance in weight-training athletes. *International Journal of Sport Nutrition*, 6: 382–390.

Fleck, S.J. (1983) Bridging the gap: Interval training physiological basis. *NSCA Journal*, 5: 57–62.

Fleming, J. et al. (2003). Endurance capacity and high-intensity exercise performance responses to a high-fat diet. *International Journal of Sport Nutrition and Exercise Metabolism*, 13: 466–478.

Foster-Powell, K., Holt, S.H.A., & Brand-Miller, J.C. (2002). International table of glycemic index and glycemic load values: 2002. *American Journal of Clinical Nutrition*, 76: 5–56.

Fry, A.C. et al. (1997). The effects of gamma-oryzanol supplementation during resistive exercise training. *International Journal of Sport Nutrition*, 7: 318–329.

Gaitanos, G.C. et al. (1991). Repeated bouts of sprint running after induced alkalosis. *Journal of Sports Science*, 9: 355–370.

Gallagher, P.M. et al. (2000). Beta-hydroxy-beta-methylbutyrate ingestion, Part I: Effects on strength and fat-free mass. *Medicine and Science in Sports and Exercise*, 32: 2109–2115.

Galloway, S.D. et al. (1996). The effects of acute phosphate supplementation in subjects of different aerobic fitness levels. *European Journal of Applied Physiology*, 72: 224–230.

Gambelunghe, C. et al. (2003). Effects of chrysin on urinary testosterone levels in human males. *Journal of Medicinal Food*, 6: 387–390.

Gao, J.P. et al. (1988). Sodium bicarbonate ingestion improves performance in interval swimming. *European Journal of Applied Physiology*, 58: 171–174.

Gaudard, A. et al. (2003). Drugs for increasing oxygen transport and their potential use in doping. *Sports Medicine*, 33: 187–212.

Gill, N.D., Hall, R.D., & Blazevich, A.J. (2004). Creatine serum is not as effective as creatine powder for improving cycle sprint performance in competitive male team-sport athletes. *Journal of Strength and Conditioning Research*, 18: 272–275.

Gill, N.D. et al. (2000). Muscular and cardiorespiratory effects of pseudoephedrine in human athletes. *British Journal of Clinical Pharmacology*, 50: 205–213.

Gillies, H. et al. (1996). Pseudoephedrine is without ergogenic effects during prolonged exercise. *Journal of Applied Physiology*, 81: 2611–2617.

Goldfinch, J., McNaughton, L. & Davies, P. (1988). Induced metabolic alkalosis and its effects on 400-m racing time. *European Journal of Applied Physiology*, 57: 45–48.

Goulet, E.D. & Dionne, I.J. (2005). Assessment of the effects of eleutherococcus senticosus on endurance performance. *International Journal of Sport Nutrition and Exercise Metabolism*, 15: 75–83.

Goworth, H.W. et al. (1997). Persistence of supercompensated muscle glycogen in trained subjects after carbohydrate loading. *Journal of Applied Physiology*, 82: 342–347.

Green, A.L. et al. (1996). Carbohydrate feeding augments skeletal muscle creatine accumulation during creatine supplementation in humans. *American Journal of Physiology*, 271: E821–E826.

Green, N.R. & Ferrando, A.A. (1994). Plasma boron and the effects of boron supplementation in males. *Environmental Health Perspectives*, 102 (suppl.): 73–77.

Greenhaff, P.L. (1996). Creatine supplementation: Recent developments. *British Journal of Sports Medicine*, 30: 276–277.

Greenwood, M. et al. (2003). Cramping and injury incidence in collegiate football players are reduced by creatine supplementation. *Journal of Athletic Training*, 38: 216–219.

Greer, F., McLean, C., & Graham, T.E. (1998). Caffeine, performance, and metabolism during repeated Wingate exercise tests. *Journal of Applied Physiology*, 85: 1502–1508

Gruber, A.J. & Pope, H.G. (1998). Ephedrine use among 36 female weightlifters. *American Journal of Addiction*, 7: 256–261.

Guerrero-Ontiveros, M.L. & Wallimann, T. (1998). Creatine supplementation in health and disease: Effects of chronic creatine ingestion in vivo: Down-regulation of the expression of creatine transporter isoforms in skeletal muscle. *Molecular and Cellular Biochemistry*, 184: 427–437.

Guilland, J.C. et al. (1989). Vitamin status of young athletes including the effects of supplementation. *Medicine and Science in Sports and Exercise*, 21: 441–449.

Ha, E. & Zemel, M.B. (2003). Functional properties of whey, whey components, and essential amino acids: Mechanisms underlying health benefits for active people. *Journal of Nutritional Biochemistry,*. 14: 251–258.

Haller, C.A., Jacob, P., & Benowitz, N.L. (2004). Enhanced stimulant and metabolic effects of combined ephedrine and caffeine. *Clinical Pharmacology and Therapeutics,* 75: 259–273.

Haller, C.A. et al. (2004). Concentrations of ephedra alkaloids and caffeine in commercial dietary supplements. *Journal of Analytical Toxicology,* 28: 145–151.

Harris, R.C., Soderlund, K., & Hultman, E. (1992). Elevation in creatine in resting and exercised muscle of normal subjects by creatine supplementation. *Clinical Science,* 83: 367–374.

Hawley, J.A., Palmer, G.S., & Noakes, T.D. (1997). Effects of three days of carbohydrate supplementation on muscle glycogen content and utilization during a 1-h cycling performance. *European Journal of Applied Physiology,* 75: 407–412.

Hawley, J.A. et al. (1997). Carbohydrate loading and exercise performance: An update. *Sports Medicine,* 24: 73–81.

Haymes, E.M. (1991). Vitamin and mineral supplementation to athletes. *International Journal of Sports Nutrition,* 1: 146–169.

Healy, M.L. et al. (2003). High dose growth hormone exerts an anabolic effect at rest and during exercise in endurance-trained athletes. *Journal of Clinical Endocrinology and Metabolism,* 88: 5221–5226.

Helge, J.W. (2000). Adaptations to a fat-rich diet: Effects on endurance performance in humans. *Sports Medicine,* 30: 347–357.

Hellsten, Y., Skadhauge, L., & Bangsbo, J. (2004). Effect of ribose supplementation on resynthesis of adenine nucleotides after immense intermittent training in humans. American *Journal of Physiology: Regulatory, Integrative and Comparative Physiology,* 286: R182–R188.

Hespel, P., Op 't eijnde, B., & Van Leemputte, M. (2002). Opposite actions of caffeine and creatine on muscle relaxation time in humans. *Journal of Applie Physiology,* 92: 513–518.

Hill, S., Box, W. & Di Silvestro, R.A. (2004). Moderate-intensity resistance exercise, plus or minus soy intake: Effects on serum lipid peroxides in young adult males. International Journal of *Sport Nutrition and Exercise Metabolism,* 14: 125–132.

Hofman, Z. et al. (2002). The effect of bovine colostrum supplementation on exercise performance in elite field hockey players. *International Journal of Sport Nutrition and Exercise Metabolism*, 12: 461–469.

Hoffman, J.R. & Falvo, M.J. (2004). Protein: Which is best? *Journal of Sports Science and Medicine*, 3: 118–130.

Hoffman, J.R. & Ratamess, N.A. (2006). Medical issues associated with anabolic steroid use: Are they exaggerated? *Journal of Sports Science and Medicine*, 5: 182–193.

Hoffman, J.R. et al. (2004). Effects of beta-hydroxy beta-methylbutyrate on power performance and indices of muscle damage and stress during high-intensity training. *Journal of Strength and Conditioning Research*, 18: 747–752.

Hongu, N. & Sachan, D.S. (2000). Caffeine, carnitine, and choline supplementation of rats decreases body fat and serum leptin concentrations as does exercise. *Journal of Nutrition*, 130: 152–157.

Horowitz, J.F. et al. (2000). Preexercise medium-chain triglyceride ingestion does not alter muscle glycogen use during exercise. *Journal of Applied Physiology*, 88: 219–225.

Horswill, C.A. et al. (1988). Influence of sodium bicarbonate on sprint performance: Relationship to dosage. *Medicine and Science in Sports and Exercise*, 20: 566–569.

Horvath, P.J. et al. (2000). The effects of varying dietary fat on performance and metabolism in trained male and female runners. *Journal of the American College of Nutrition*, 19: 52–60.

Ivy, J.L. (1998). Effect of pyruvate and dihydroxyacetone on metabolism and aerobic endurance capacity. *Medicine and Science in Sports and Exercise*, 30: 837–843.

Jacobs, I., Pasternak, H., & Bell, D.G. (2003). Effects of ephedrine, caffeine, and their combination on muscular endurance. *Medicine and Science in Sports and Exercise*, 35: 987–994.

Jacobson, B.H. & Edwards, S.W. (1991). Influence of two levels of caffeine on maximal torque at selected angular velocities. *Journal of Sports Medicine and Physical Fitness*, 31: 147–153.

Jacobson, B.H. et al. (1992). Effect of caffeine on maximal strength and power in elite male athletes. British Journal of Sports Medicine, 26: 276–280.

Jeukendrup, A.E. & Aldred, S. (2004). Fat supplementation, health, and endurance performance. *Nutrition*, 20: 678–688.

Jeukendrup, A.E. et al. (1998). Effect of medium-chain triacylglycerol and carbohydrate ingestion during exercise on substrate utilization and subsequent cycling performance. *American Journal of Clinical Nutrition*, 67: 397–404.

Jezova, D., Komadel, L., & Mikulaj, L. (1987). Plasma testosterone response to repeated human chorionic gonadotropin administration is increased in trained athletes. *Endocrinologia Experimentalis*, 21: 143–147.

Jowko, E. et al. (2001). Creatine and beta-hydroxy-beta-methylbutyrate (HMB) additively increase lean body mass and muscle strength during a weight-training program. *Nutrition*, 17: 558–566.

Kalman, D. et al. (1999). The effects of pyruvate supplementation on body composition in overweight individuals. *Nutrition*, 15: 337–340.

Kanayama, G. et al. (2001). Over-the-counter drug use in gymnasiums: An unrecognized substance abuse problem? *Psychotherapy and Psychosomatics*, 70: 137–140.

Karch, S.B. (2002). *Amphetamines. In: Performance-Enhancing Substances in Sport and Exercise* (Eds. M.S. Bahrke & C.E. Yesalis). Champaign, IL: Human Kinetics, pp. 257–265.

Karila, T.A. et al. (2003). Anabolic androgenic steroids produce dose-dependant increase in left ventricular mass in power athletes, and this effect is potentiated by concomitant use of growth hormone. *International Journal of Sports Medicine*, 24: 337–343.

Karlic, H. & Lohninger, A. (2004). Supplementation of L-carnitine in athletes: Does it make sense? *Nutrition*, 20: 709–715.

Kellis, J.T. & Vickery, L.E. (1984). Inhibition of human estrogen synthetase (aromatase) by flavones. *Science*, 225: 1032–1034.

Kelly, G.S. (2001). Conjugated linoleic acid: A review. *Alternative Medicine Review*, 6: 367–382.

Kilduff, L.P. et al. (2004). The effects of creatine supplementation on cardiovascular, metabolic, and thermoregulatory responses during exercise in the heat in endurance-trained men. *International Journal of Sport Nutrition and Exercise Metabolism*, 14: 443–460.

Kim, H. et al. (2003). Octacosanol supplementation increases running endurance time and improves biochemical parameters after exhaustion in trained rats. *Journal of Medicinal Food*, 6: 345–351.

King, D.S. et al. (1999). Effect of oral androstenedione on serum testosterone and adaptations to resistance training in young men: A randomized controlled trial. *Journal of the American Medical Association*, 281: 2020–2028.

Kleiner, S.M. & Greenwood-Robinson, M. (2001). *Power Eating*, 2nd ed. Champaign, IL: Human Kinetics.

Knitter, A.E. et al. (2000). Effects of beta-hydroxy-beta-methylbutyrate on muscle damage after a prolonged run. *Journal of Applied Physiology*, 89: 1340–1344.

Koh-Banerjee, P.K. et al. (2005). Effects of calcium pyruvate supplementation during training on body composition, exercise capacity, and metabolic responses to exercise. *Nutrition*, 21: 312–319.

Kohut, M.L. et al. (2003). Ingestion of a dietary supplement containing dehydroepiandrosterone (DHEA) and androstenedione has minimal effect on immune function in middle-aged men. *Journal of the American College of Nutrition*, 22: 363–371.

Kolkhorst, F.W. et al. (2004). Effects of sodium bicarbonate on $\dot{V}O_2$ kinetics during heavy exercise. *Medicine and Science in Sports and Exercise*, 36: 1895–1899.

Kozak-Collins, K., Burke, E.R., & Schoene, R.B. (1994). Sodium bicarbonate ingestion does not improve performance in women cyclists. *Medicine and Science in Sports and Exercise*, 26: 1510–1515.

Kraemer, W.J., Nindl, B.C., & Rubin, M.R. (2002). Growth hormone: Physiological effects of exogenous administration. In: *Performance-Enhancing Substances in Sport and Exercise* (Eds. M.S. Bahrke & C.E. Yesalis). Champaign, IL: Human Kinetics, pp. 65–78.

Kraemer, W.J. et al. (2005). Cortitrol supplementation reduces serum cortisol responses to physical stress. *Metabolism*, 54: 657–668.

Kraemer, W.J. et al. (2005). Body size and composition of National Football League players. *Journal of Strength and Conditioning Research*, 19: 485–489.

Kraemer, W.J. et al. (2003). The effects of L-carnitine L-tartrate supplementation on hormonal responses to resistance exercise and recovery. *Journal of Strength and Conditioning Research*, 17: 455–462.

Kraemer, W.J. et al. (1995). Effects of multibuffer supplementation on acid-base balance and 2,3-diphosphoglycerate following repetitive anaerobic exercise. *International Journal of Sport Nutrition*, 5: 300–314.

Kreider, R.B. et al. (2003). Long-term creatine supplementation does not significantly affect clinical markers of health in athletes. Molecular and Cellular Biochemistry, 244: 95–104.

Kreider, R.B. et al. (2003). Effects of oral D-ribose supplementation on anaerobic capacity and selected metabolic markers in healthy males. *International Journal of Sport Nutrition*, 13: 87–96.

Kreider, R.B. et al. (2002). Effects of conjugated linoleic acid supplementation during resistance training on body composition, bone density, strength, and selected hematological markers. *Journal of Strength and Conditioning Research*, 16: 325–334.

Kreider, R.B. et al. (1999). Effects of calcium beta-hydroxy-beta-methylbutyrate (HMB) supplementation during resistance-training on markers of catabolism, body composition and strength. *International Journal of Sports Medicine*, 20: 503–509.

Kreider, R.B. et al. (1992). Effects of phosphate loading on metabolic and myocardial responses to maximal and endurance exercise. *International Journal of Sports Nutrition*, 2: 20–47.

Kreider, R.B. et al. (1990). Effects of phosphate loading on oxygen uptake, ventilatory anaerobic threshold, and run performance. *Medicine and Science in Sports and Exercise*, 22: 250–256.

Kriketos, A.D. (1999). (-)-Hydroxycitric acid does not affect energy expenditure and substrate oxidation in adult males in a post-absorptive state. *International Journal of Obesity-Related Metabolic Disorders*, 23: 867–873.

Kumar, N. et al. (1999). 7 alpha-methyl-19-nortestosterone, a synthetic androgen with high potency: Structure-activity comparisons with other androgens. *Journal of Steroid Biochemistry and Molecular Biology*, 71: 213–222.

La Botz, M. & Smith, B.W. (1999). Creatine supplement use in an NCAA Division I athletic program. *Clinical Journal of Sports Medicine*, 9: 167–169.

Labrie, F. et al. (1997). Physiological changes in dehydroepiandrosterone are not reflected by serum levels of active androgens and estrogens but of their metabolites: Intracrinology. *Journal of Clinical Endocrinology and Metabolism*, 82: 2403–2409.

Laskowski, R. & Antosiewicz, J. (2003). Increased adaptability of young judo sportsmen after protein supplementation. *Journal of Sports Medicine and Physical Fitness*, 43: 342–346.

Lavender, G. & Bird, S.R. (1989). Effect of sodium bicarbonate ingestion upon repeated sprints. *British Journal of Sports Medicine*, 23: 41–45.

Le Boucher, J. et al. (1997). Enteral administration of ornithine alpha-ketoglutarate or arginine alpha-ketoglutarate: a comparative study of their effects on glutamine pools in burn-injured rats. *Critical Care Medicine*, 25: 293–298.

Leder, B.Z. et al. (2000) Oral androstenedione administration and serum testosterone concentrations in young men. *Journal of the American Medical Association*, 283: 779–782.

Lehmkuhl, M. et al. (2003). The effects of 8 weeks of creatine monohydrate and glutamine supplementation on body composition and performance measures. *Journal of Strength and Conditioning Research*, 17: 425–438.

Leigh-Smith, S. (2004). Blood boosting. *British Journal of Sports Medicine*, 38: 99–101.

Lemon, P.W.R. (1987). Protein and exercise: Update 1987. *Medicine and Science in Sports and Exercise*, 19 (suppl.): S179–S190

Lemon, P.W.R. et al. (1992). Protein requirements and muscle mass/strength changes during intensive training in novice bodybuilders. *Journal of Applied Physiology*, 73: 767–775.

Liang, M.T., Podolka, T.D., & Chuang, W.J. (2005). Panax notoginseng supplementation enhances physical performance during endurance exercise. *Journal of Strength and Conditioning Research*, 19: 108–114.

Lim, K. et al. (2003). (-)-Hydroxycitric acid ingestion increases fat utilization during exercise in untrained women. *Journal of Nutritional Vitaminology (Tokyo)*, 49: 163–167.

Lim, K. et al. (2002). Short-term (-)-hydroxycitrate ingestion increases fat oxidation during exercise in athletes. *Journal of Nutritional Vitaminology (Tokyo)*, 48: 128–133.

Livolsi, J.M., Adams, G.M, & Laguna, P.L. (2001). The effect of chromium picolinate on muscular strength and body composition in women athletes. *Journal of Strength and Conditioning Research*, 15: 161–166.

Llewellyn, W. (2005). *Anabolics 2005: Anabolic Steroid Reference Manual*. Jupiter, FL: Body of Science.

Lukaski, H.C. et al. (1996). Chromium supplementation and resistance training: Effects on body composition, strength, and trace element status of men. *American Journal of Clinical Nutrition*, 63: 954–965.

Lukaski, H.C. (2004). Vitamin and mineral status: Effects on physical performance. *Nutrition*, 20: 632–644, 2004.

Lynch, G.S. (2002). Beta-2 agonists. In: *Performance-Enhancing Substances in Sport and Exercise* (Eds. M.S. Bahrke & C.E. Yesalis). Champaign, IL: Human Kinetics, pp. 47–64.

MacDougall, J.D. et al. (1995). The time course for elevated muscle protein synthesis following heavy resistance exercise. *Canadian Journal of Applied Physiology*, 20: 480–486.

MacDougall, J.D. et al. (1992). Changes in muscle protein synthesis following heavy resistance exercise in humans: A pilot study. *Acta Physiologica Scandinavica*, 146: 403–404.

Magkos, F. & Kavouras, S.A. (2004). Caffeine and ephedrine: Physiological, metabolic and performance-enhancing effects. *Sports Medicine*, 34: 871–889.

Mahesh, V.B. & Greenblatt, R.B. (1962). The in vivo conversion of dehydroepiandrosterone to testosterone in the human. *Acta Endocrinologica*, 41: 400-406.

Marques-Magallanes, J.A. et al. (1997). Impact of habitual cocaine smoking on the physiologic response to maximum exercise. *Chest*, 112: 1008–1016.

Marsit, J.L., Conley, M.S., & Stone, M.H. (1993). The effect of different doses of sodium bicarbonate on performance of the leg press exercise. *Journal of Strength and Conditioning Research*, 7: 184.

Massad, S.J. et al. (1995). High school athletes and nutritional supplements: A study of knowledge and use. *International Journal of Sport Nutrition*, 5: 232–245.

Matson, L.G. & Tran, Z.V. (1993). Effects of sodium bicarbonate ingestion on anaerobic performance: A meta-analytic review. *International Journal of Sport Nutrition*, 3: 2–28.

McNaughton, L. & Cedaro, R. (1992). Sodium citrate ingestion and its effects on maximal anaerobic exercise of different durations. *European Journal of Applied Physiology*, 64: 36–41.

McNaughton, L., Egan, G., & Caelli, G. (1989). A comparison of Chinese and Russian ginseng as ergogenic aids to improve various facets of physical fitness. *International Clinical Nutrition Review*, 90: 32–35.

McNaughton, L. & Thompson, D. (2001). Acute versus chronic sodium bicarbonate ingestion and anaerobic work and power output. *Journal of Sports Medicine and Physical Fitness*, 41: 456–462.

McNaughton, L. et al. (1999). Effect of chronic bicarbonate ingestion on the performance of high-intensity work. *European Journal of Applied Physiology*, 80: 333–336.

McNaughton, L.R. (1992a). Bicarbonate ingestion: Effects of dosage on 60 s cycle ergometry. *Journal of Sports Science*, 10: 415–423.

McNaughton, L.R. (1992b). Sodium bicarbonate ingestion and its effects on anaerobic exercise of various durations. *Journal of Sports Science*, 10: 425–435.

McNaughton, L.R. (1990). Sodium citrate and anaerobic performance: implications of dosage. *European Journal of Applied Physiology*, 61: 392–397.

Mero, A. et al. (1997). Effects of bovine colostrum supplementation on serum IGF-1, IgG, hormone and saliva IgA during training. *Journal of Applied Physiology*, 93: 732–739.

Metzl, J.D. et al. (2001). Creatine use among young athletes. *Pediatrics*, 108: 421–425.

Micheletti, A., Rossi, R., & Rufini, S. (2001). Zinc status in athletes: Relation to diet and exercise. *Sports Medicine*, 31: 577–582.

Mickleborough, T.D. (2003). Fish oil supplementation reduces severity of exercise-induced bronchoconstriction in elite athletes. *American Journal of Respiratory and Critical Care Medicine*, 168: 1181–1189.

Miller, S.L. (2003). Independent and combined effects of amino acids and glucose after resistance exercise. *Medicine and Science in Sports and Exercise*, 35: 449–455.

Millington, D.S. & Dubag, G. (1993). Dietary supplement L-carnitine: Analysis of different brands to determine bioavailability and content. *Clinical Research and Regulatory Affairs*, 10: 71–80.

Morris, A.C. et al. (1996). No ergogenic effects of ginseng ingestion. *International Journal Sport Nutrition*, 6: 263–271

Morrison, M.A., Spriet, L.L., & Dyck, D.J. (2000). Pyruvate ingestion for 7 days does not improve aerobic performance in well-trained individuals. *Journal of Applied Physiology*, 89: 549–556.

Naghii, M.R. & Samman, S. (1997). The effect of boron supplementation on its urinary excretion and selected cardiovascular risk factors in healthy male subjects. *Biological Trace Element Research*, 56: 273–286.

Naghii, M.R. & Samman, S. (1993). The role of boron in nutrition and metabolism. *Progress in Food and Nutrition Science*, 17: 331–349.

Newhouse, I.J. & Finstad, E.W. (2000). The effects of magnesium supplementation on exercise performance. *Clinical Journal of Sports Medicine*, 10: 195–200.

Neychev, V.K. & Mitev, V.I. (2005). The aphrodisiac herb Tribulus terrestris does not influence the androgen production in young men. *Journal of Ethnopharmacology*, Jun 30.

Nielsen, P. & Nachtigall, D. (1998). Iron supplementation in athletes: Current recommendations. *Sports Medicine*, 26: 207–216.

Nikawa, T. et al. (2002).Effects of a soy protein diet on exercise-induced muscle protein catabolism in rats. *Nutrition*, 18: 490–495

Nissen, S. (2000). Beta-hydroxy-beta-methylbutyrate (HMB) supplementation in humans is safe and may decrease cardiovascular risk factors. *Journal of Nutrition*, 130: 1937–1945.

Nissen, S.L. & Sharp, R.L. (2003). Effect of dietary supplements on lean mass and strength gains with resistance exercise: A meta-analysis. *Journal of Applied Physiology*, 94: 651–659.

Nissen, S. et al. (1996) Effect of leucine metabolite β-hydroxy-β-methylbutyrate on muscle metabolism during resistance-exercise training. *Journal of Applied Physiology*, 81: 2095–2104.

O'Connor, D.M. & Crowe, M.J. (2003). Effects of beta-hydroxy-beta-methylbutyrate and creatine monohydrate supplementation on the aerobic and anaerobic capacity of highly trained athletes. *Journal of Sports Medicine and Physical Fitness*, 43: 64–68.

Oopik, V. (2003). (2003). Effects of sodium citrate ingestion before exercise on endurance performance in well trained college runners. *British Journal of Sports Medicine*, 37: 485–489.

Op T' Eijnde, B. et al. (2001). No effects of oral ribose supplementation on repeated maximal exercise and de novo ATP resynthesis. *Journal of Applied Physiology*, 91: 2275–2281.

Pace, N. et al. (1947). The increase in hypoxic tolerance of normal men accompanying the polycythaemia induced by transfusion of erythrocytes. *American Journal of Physiology*, 1: 152–163.

Paddon-Jones, D., Keech, A., & Jenkins, D. (2001). Short-term beta-hydroxy-beta-methylbutyrate supplementation does not reduce symptoms of eccentric muscle damage. *International Journal of Sport Nutrition and Exercise Metabolism*, 11: 442–450.

Panton, L.B. et al. (2000). Nutritional supplementation of the leucine metabolite beta-hydroxy-beta-methylbutyrate (HMB) during resistance training. *Nutrition*, 16: 734–739.

Parcell, A.C. et al. (2004). Cordyceps Sinensis (CordyMax Cs-4) supplementation does not improve endurance exercise performance. *International Journal of Sport Nutrition and Exercise Metabolism*, 14: 236–242

Parisotto, R. et al. (2001). Detection of recombinant human erythropoietin abuse in athletes utilizing markers of altered erythropoiesis. *Haematologica*, 86: 128–137

Parkinson, A.B. & Evans, N.A. (2006). Anabolic androgenic steroids: A survey of 500 users. *Medicine and Science in Sports and Exercise*, 38: 644–651.

Parry-Billings, M. & MacLaren, D.P. (1986). The effect of sodium bicarbonate and sodium citrate ingestion on anaerobic power during intermittent exercise. *European Journal of Applied Physiology*, 55: 524–529.

Paul, D.R. et al. (2001). Carbohydrate-loading during the follicular phase of the menstrual cycle: Effects on muscle glycogen and exercise performance. *International Journal of Sport Nutrition and Exercise Metabolism*, 11: 430–441.

Pendergast, D., Leddy, J.J., & Venkatraman, J.T. (2000) A perspective on fat intake in athletes. *Journal of the American College of Nutrition*, 19: 345–350.

Perry, P.J. et al. (2005).Anabolic steroid use in weightlifters and bodybuilders: An internet survey of drug utilization. *Clinical Journal of Sport Medicine*, 15: 326–330.

Phillips, S.M. et al. (1999) Resistance training reduces the acute exercise-induced increase in muscle protein turnover. *American Journal of Physiology: Endocrinology and Metabolism*, 276: E118–E124.

Phillips, S.M. et al. (1997). Mixed muscle protein synthesis and breakdown after resistance exercise in humans. *American Journal of Physiology: Endocrinology and Metabolism*, 273: E99–E107.

Pittler, M.H. & Ernst, E. (2004). Dietary supplements for body-weight reduction: A systematic review. *American Journal of Clinical Nutrition*, 79: 529–536.

Portington, K.J. et al. (1998). Effect of induced alkalosis on exhaustive leg press performance. *Medicine and Science in Sports and Exercise*, 30: 523–528.

Potteiger, J.A. et al. (1996). Sodium citrate ingestion enhances 30 km cycling performance. *International Journal of Sports Medicine*, 17: 7–11.

Prather, I.D. et al. (1995). Clenbuterol: A substitute for anabolic steroids? *Medicine and Science in Sports and Exercise*, 27: 1118–1121.

Preuss, H.G. et al. (2002). Citrus aurantium as a thermogenic, weight-reduction replacement for ephedra: An overview. *Journal of Medicine*, 33: 247–264.

Raastad, T., Hostmark, A.T., & Stromme, S.B. (1997). Omega-3 fatty acid supplementation does not improve maximal aerobic power, anaerobic threshold and running performance in well-trained soccer players. *Scandinavian Journal of Medicine and Science in Sports* 7: 25–31.

Ransone, J. (2003). The effect of beta-hydroxy beta-methylbutyrate on muscular strength and body composition in collegiate football players. *Journal of Strength and Conditioning Research*, 17: 34–39.

Ratamess, N.A. (2004). Amino acid supplementation: What can it really do for you? *Pure Power*, 4: 38–42.

Ratamess, N.A. et al. (2005). Effects of heavy resistance exercise volume on post-exercise androgen receptor content in resistance-trained men. *Journal of Steroid Biochemistry and Molecular Biology*, 93: 35–42.

Ratamess, N.A. et al. (2003). The effects of amino acid supplementation on muscular performance during resistance training overreaching: Evidence of an effective overreaching protocol. *Journal of Strength and Conditioning Research*, 17: 250–258.

Rauch, L.H. et al. (1995). The effects of carbohydrate loading on muscle glycogen content and cycling performance. *International Journal of Sport Nutrition*, 5: 25–36.

Rawson, E.S. & Clarkson, P.M. (2002). Ephedrine as an ergogenic aid. In: *Performing-Enhancing Substances in Sport and Exercise* (Eds. M.S. Bahrke & C.E. Yesalis). Champaign, IL: Human Kinetics, pp. 289–298.

Rawson, E.S. & Volek, J.S. (2003). Effects of creatine supplementation and resistance training on muscle strength and weightlifting performance. *Journal of Strength and Conditioning Research*, 17: 822–831.

Requena, B. et al. (2005). Sodium bicarbonate and sodium citrate: Ergogenic aids. *Journal of Strength and Conditioning Research*, 19: 213–224.

Rodriguez-Melendez, R. & Zempleni, J. (2003). Regulation of gene expression by biotin. *Journal of Nutritional Biochemistry*, 14: 680–690.

Rosene, J.M., Whitman, S.A. & Fogarty, T.D. (2004). A comparison of thermoregulation with creatine supplementation between the sexes in a thermoneutral environment. *Journal of Athletic Training*, 39: 50–55.

Rubin, M.R. et al. (2001). Safety measures of L-carnitine L-tartrate supplementation in healthy men. *Journal of Strength and Conditioning Research*, 15: 486–490.

Russell, G. et al. (2002). Effects of prolonged low doses of recombinant human erythropoietin during submaximal and maximal exercise. *European Journal of Applied Physiology*, 86: 442–449.

Sachan, D.S. & Hongu, N. (2000). Increases in $\dot{V}O_2$ max and metabolic markers of fat oxidation by caffeine, carnitine, and choline supplementation in rats. *Journal of Nutritional Biochemistry*, 11: 521–526.

Saint-John, M. & McNaughton, L. (1986). Octacosanol ingestion and its effects on metabolic responses to submaximal cycle ergometry, reaction time and chest and grip strength. *International Clinical Nutrition Review*, 6: 81–87.

Sanguineti, V.R. & Frank, M.R. (2002). Gamma-hydroxybutyric acid. In: *Performance-Enhancing Substances in Sport and Exercise* (Eds. M.S. Bahrke & C.E. Yesalis). Champaign, IL: Human Kinetics, pp. 299–304.

Sawka, M.N. et al. (1987). Erythrocyte reinfusion and maximal aerobic power: An examination of modifying factors. *Journal of the American Medical Association*, 257: 1496–1499.

Selsby, J.T., DiSilvestro, R.A., & Devor, S.T. (2004). Mg++-creatine chelate and a low-dose creatine supplementation regimen improve exercise performance. *Journal of Strength and Conditioning Research*, 18: 311–315.

Shafat, A. et al. (2004). Effects of dietary supplementation with vitamins C and E on muscle function during and after eccentric contractions in humans. *European Journal of Applied Physiology*, 93: 196–202.

Shave, R. et al. (2001). The effects of sodium citrate ingestion on 3,000-meter time-trial performance. *Journal of Strength and Conditioning Research*, 15: 230–234.

Shekelle, P.G. et al. (2003). Efficacy and safety of ephedra and ephedrine for weight loss and athletic performance: A meta-analysis. *Journal of the American Medical Association*, 289: 1537–1545.

Slater, G. et al. (2001). Beta-hydroxy-beta-methylbutyrate (HMB) supplementation does not affect changes in strength or body composition during resistance training in trained men. *International Journal of Sport Nutrition and Exercise Metabolism*, 11: 384–396.

Soares, M.J. et al. (1993). The effect of exercise on the riboflavin status of adult men. *British Journal of Nutrition*, 69: 541–551.

Sobal, J. & Marquart, L.F. (1994). Vitamin/mineral supplement use among athletes: A review of the literature. *International Journal of Sport Nutrition*, 4: 320–334.

Soop, M. et al. (1988). Influence of carnitine supplementation on muscle substrate and carnitine metabolism during exercise. *Journal of Applied Physiology*, 64: 2394–2399.

Spector, S.A. et al. (1995). Effect of choline supplementation on fatigue in trained cyclists. *Medicine and Science in Sports and Exercise*, 27: 668–673.

Spriet, L.L. (2002). Caffeine. In: *Performance-Enhancing Substances in Sport and Exercise* (Eds. M.S. Bahrke & C.E. Yesalis). Champaign, IL: Human Kinetics, pp. 267–278.

Stainback, R.D. & Cohen, R.J. (2002). Alcohol use in sport and exercise. In: *Performance-Enhancing Substances in Sport and Exercise* (Eds. M.S. Bahrke & C.E. Yesalis). Champaign, IL: Human Kinetics, pp. 227–245.

Stanko, R.T. et al. (1990a). Enhancement of arm exercise endurance capacity with dihydroxyacetone and pyruvate. *Journal of Applied Physiology*, 68: 119–124.

Stanko, R.T. et al. (1990b). Enhanced leg exercise endurance with a high-carbohydrate diet and dihydroxyacetone and pyruvate. *Journal of Applied Physiology*, 69: 1651–1656.

Starling, R.D. et al. (1997). Effects of diet on muscle triglyceride and endurance performance. *Journal of Applied Physiology*, 82: 1185–1189.

Stone, M.H. et al. (1999). Effects of in-season (5 weeks) creatine and pyruvate supplementation on anaerobic performance and body composition in American football players. *International Journal of Sport Nutrition*, 9: 146–165.

Suzuki, Y. et al. (2002). High level of skeletal muscle carnosine contributes to the latter half of exercise performance during 30-s maximal cycle ergometer sprinting. Japanese *Journal of Physiology*, 52: 199–205.

Stewart, I. et al. (1990). Phosphate loading and the effects on $\dot{V}O_2$ max in trained cyclists. *Research Quarterly for Exercise and Sport*, 61: 80–84.

Swain, R.A. et al. (1997). Do pseudoephedrine or phenylpropanolamine improve maximum oxygen uptake and time to exhaustion? *Clinical Journal of Sports Medicine*, 7: 168–173.

Syrotuik, D.G. & Bell, G.J. (2004). Acute creatine monohydrate supplementation: A descriptive physiological profile of responders and nonresponders. *Journal of Strength and Conditioning Research*, 18: 610–617.

Takanami, Y. et al. (2000). Vitamin E supplementation and endurance exercise: Are there benefits? *Sports Medicine*, 29: 73–83.

Tarnopolsky, M. et al. (2003). Acute and moderate-term creatine monohydrate supplementation does not affect creatine transporter mRNA or protein content in either young or elderly humans. *Molecular and Cellular Biochemistry*, 244: 159–166.

Tarnopolsky, M.A. et al. (1992). Evaluation of protein requirements for trained strength athletes. *Journal of Applied Physiology*, 73: 1986–1995.

Taylor, W.N. (2002). *Anabolic Steroids and the Athlete*, 2nd ed. Jefferson, NC: McFarland and Co.

Thomson, J.S. (2004). Beta-hydroxy-beta-methylbutyrate (HMB) supplementation of resistance trained men. *Asia Pacific Journal of Clinical Nutrition*, 13(suppl.): S59.

Tipton, K.D. et al. (2003). Acute response of net muscle protein balance reflects 24-h balance after exercise and amino acid ingestion. *American Journal of Physiology: Endocrinology and Metabolism*, 284: E76–E89.

Tipton, K.D. et al. (2001). Timing of amino acid-carbohydrate ingestion alters anabolic response of muscle to resistance exercise. *American Journal of Physiology: Endocrinology and Metabolism*, 281: E197–E206.

Tipton, K.D. et al. (1999). Postexercise net protein synthesis in human muscle from orally administered amino acids. *American Journal of Physiology: Endocrinology and Metabolism*, 276: E628–E634.

Tiryaki, G.R. & Atterbom, H.A. (1995). The effects of sodium bicarbonate and sodium citrate on 600 m running time of trained females. *Journal of Sports Medicine and Physical Fitness*, 35: 194–198.

Tomita, K. et al. (2003). (-)-Hydroxycitrate ingestion increases fat oxidation during moderate intensity exercise in untrained men. *Bioscience, Biotechnology and Biochemechanics*, 67: 1999–2001.

Tseng, Y.L. et al. (2003). Ephedrines in over-the-counter cold medicines and urine specimens collected during sport competitions. *Journal of Analytical Toxicology*, 27: 359–365.

Uralets, V.P. & Gillette, P.A. (1999). Over-the-counter anabolic steroids 4-androsten-3,17-dione; 4-androsten-3beta,17beta-diol; and 19-nor-4-androsten-3,17-dione: Excretion studies in men. *Journal of Analytical Toxicology*, 23: 357–366.

Van Blitterswijk, W.J., van de Nes, J.C.S., & Wuisman, P.I.J.M. (2003). Glucosamine and chondroitin sulfate supplementation to treat symptomatic disc generation: biochemical rationale and case report. *BMC Complementary and Alternative Medicine*, 3: 1–8.

Van Gammeren, D., Falk, D., & Antonio, J. (2002). Effects of norandrostenedione and norandrostenediol in resistance-trained men. *Nutrition*, 18: 734–737.

Van Gammeren, D., Falk, D., & Antonio, J. (2001). The effects of supplementation with 19-nor-4-androstene-3,17-dione and 19-nor-4-androstene-3,17-diol on body composition and athletic performance in previously weight-trained male athletes. *European Journal of Applied Physiology*, 84: 426–431.

Van Loon, L.J.C. et al. (2000). Effects of acute (-)-hydroxycitrate supplementation on substrate metabolism at rest and during exercise in humans. *American Journal of Clinical Nutrition*, 72: 1445–1450.

Van Montfoort, M.C.E. et al. (2004). Effects of ingestion of bicarbonate, citrate, lactate, and chloride on sprint running. *Medicine and Science in Sports and Exercise*, 36: 1239–1243.

Van Someren, K. et al. (1998). An investigation into the effects of sodium citrate ingestion on high-intensity exercise performance. *International Journal of Sports Nutrition*, 8: 356–363.

Van Zant, R.S., Conway, J.M., & Seale, J.L. (2002). A moderate carbohydrate and fat diet does not impair strength performance in moderately trained males. *Journal of Sports Medicine and Physical Fitness*, 42: 31–37.

Vandenberghe, K. et al. (1996). Caffeine counteracts the ergogenic action of muscle creatine loading. *Journal of Applied Physiology*, 80: 452–457.

Viitala, P. & Newhouse, I.J. (2004). Vitamin E supplementation, exercise and lipid peroxidation in human participants. *European Journal of Applied Physiology*, 93: 108–115.

Vincent, J.B. (2003). The potential value and toxicity of chromium picolinate as a nutritional supplement, weight loss agent and muscle development agent. *Sports Medicine*, 33: 213–230.

Vogt, M. et al. (2003). Effects of dietary fat on muscle substrates, metabolism, and performance in athletes. *Medicine and Science in Sports and Exercise*, 35: 952–960.

Volek, J.S. (2003). Strength nutrition. *Current Sports Medicine Reports*, 2: 189–193.

Volek, J.S. & Rawson, E.S. (2004). Scientific basis and practical aspects of creatine supplementation for athletes. *Nutrition*, 20: 609–614.

Volek, J.S. et al. (2004). The effects of creatine supplementation on muscular performance and body composition responses to short-term resistance training overreaching. *European Journal of Applied Physiology*, 91: 628–637.

Volek, J.S. et al. (2002). L-Carnitine L-tartrate supplementation favorably affects markers of recovery from exercise stress. *American Journal of Physiology: Endocrinology and Metabolism*, 282: E474–E482.

Vukovich, M.D., Costill, D.L., & Fink, W.J. (1994). Carnitine supplementation: effect on muscle carnitine and glycogen content during exercise. *Medicine and Science in Sports and Exercise*, 26: 1122–1129.

Vukovich, M.D., Stubbs, N.B., & Bohlken, R.M. (2001). Body composition in 70-year-old adults responds to dietary beta-hydroxy-beta-methylbutyrate similarly to that of young adults. *Journal of Nutrition*, 131: 2049–2052.

Wagenmakers, A.J.M. (1999). Amino acid supplements to improve athletic performance. *Current Opinion in Clinical Nutrition and Metabolic Care*, 2: 539–544.

Walker, L.S. et al. (1998). Chromium picolinate effects on body composition and muscular performance in wrestlers. *Medicine and Science in Sports and Exercise*, 30: 1730–1737.

Wallace, M.B. et al. (1999). Effects of dehydroepiandrosterone vs androstenedione supplementation in men. *Medicine and Science in Sports and Exercise*, 31: 1788–1792.

Walzel, B. et al. (2002). New creatine transporter assay and identification of distinct creatine transporter isoforms in muscle. *American Journal of Physiology: Endocrinology and Metabolism*, 283: E390–E401.

Wang, Y. & Jones, P.J.H. (2004). Dietary conjugated linoleic acid and body composition. *American Journal of Clinical Nutrition*, 79 (suppl.): 1153S–1158S.

Warber, J.P. et al. (2000). The effects of choline supplementation on physical performance. *International Journal of Sports Nutrition and Exercise Metabolism*, 10: 170–181.

Watsford, M.L. et al. (2003). Creatine supplementation and its effect on musculotendinous stiffness and performance. *Journal of Strength and Conditioning Research*, 17: 26–33.

Watson, G. et al. (2005). Influence of diuretic-induced dehydration on competitive sprint and power performance. *Medicine and Science in Sports and Exercise*, 37: 1168–1174.

Watt, K.K., Garnham, A.P., & Snow, R.J. (2004). Skeletal muscle total creatine content and creatine transporter gene expression in vegetarians prior to and following creatine supplementation. *International Journal of Sports Nutrition and Exercise Metabolism*, 14: 517–531.

Weber, M.M. (2002). Effects of growth hormone on skeletal muscle. *Hormone Research*, 3(suppl.): 43–48.

Webster, M.J. (1999). Sodium bicarbonate. In: *Performing-Enhancing Substances in Sport and Exercise*. (Eds. M.S. Bahrke & C.E. Yesalis). Champaign, IL: Human Kinetics, pp. 197–207.

Webster, M.J. et al. (1993). Effect of sodium bicarbonate ingestion on exhaustive resistance exercise performance. *Medicine and Science in Sports and Exercise*, 25: 960–965.

Wilkes, D., Gledhill, N., & Smyth, R. (1983). Effect of acute induced metabolic alkalosis on 800-m racing time. *Medicine and Science in Sports and Exercise*, 15: 277–280.

Williams, A.G. et al. (2001). Is glucose/amino acid supplementation after exercise an aid to strength training? *British Journal of Sports Medicine*, 35: 109–113.

Williams, M.H. (1999). Facts and fallacies of purported ergogenic amino acid supplements. *Clinical Sports Medicine*, 18: 633–649.

Williams, M.H. (1998). *The Ergogenics Edge*. Champaign, IL: Human Kinetics.

Williams, M.H. et al. (1981). The effect of induced erythrocythemia upon 5-mile treadmill run time. *Medicine and Science in Sports and Exercise*, 13: 169–175.

Williams, M.H., Kreider, R.B., & Branch, J.D. (1999). *Creatine: The power supplement*. Champaign, IL: Human Kinetics.

Willoughby, D.S. (2004). Effects of an alleged myostatin-binding supplement and heavy resistance training on serum myostatin, muscle strength and mass, and body composition. *International Journal of Sports Nutrition and Exercise Metabolism*, 14: 461–472.

Winters-Stone, K.M. & Snow, C.M. (2004). One year of oral calcium supplementation maintains cortical bone density in young adult female distance runners. *International Journal of Sports Nutrition and Exercise Metabolism*, 14: 7–17.

Yesails, C.E. et al. (2000). Incidence of anabolic steroid use: A discussion of methodological issues. In: *Anabolic Steroids in Sports & Exercise*, 2nd ed. Champaign, IL: Human Kinetics,1 pp. 73–115.

Yoshizumi, W.M. & Tsourounis, C. (2004). Effects of creatine supplementation on renal function. *Journal of Herbal Pharmacotherapy*, 4: 1–7.

Zoller, H. & Vogel, W. (2004) Iron supplementation in athletes—first do no harm. *Nutrition*, 20: 615–619.

About the Author

Nicholas A. Ratamess, Ph.D., CSCS*D, is an assistant professor in the department of Health and Exercise Science at The College of New Jersey.

A former fitness instructor, strength coach, and competitive power lifter who earned a Ph.D. in kinesiology from the University of Connecticut, Dr. Ratamess's major research interest is examining how the human body physiologically adapts to resistance training and how performance can be optimized through resistance training and supplementation.

Dr. Ratamess has authored or coauthored more than 60 scientific investigations, educational articles, review papers, and book chapters on strength and conditioning and sports supplementation. He is a Certified Strength and Conditioning Specialist with Distinction and a USA Weightlifting Level I Club Coach who is an active member of the National Strength and Conditioning Association, American College of Sports Medicine, and International Society of Biomechanics in Sports.